Psoriasis

The Real Way Out

A Self-Education Guide
For Complete Natural Healing

Psoriasis

The Real Way Out

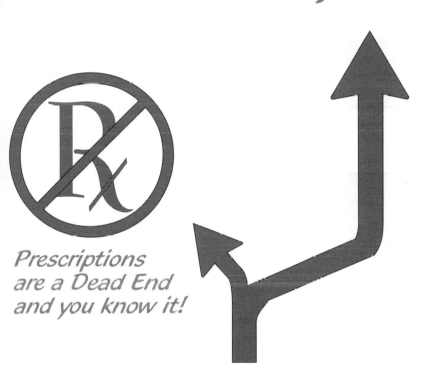

*Prescriptions
are a Dead End
and you know it!*

A Self-Education Guide for Complete Natural Healing

Jerry G. Scott

ISBN 1-55056-958-9

Published by Jerry G. Scott
For ordering information, contact:
The Psoriasis Connection
P.O. Box 1050
Kenora, Ontario, Canada P9N 3X7
Order online at www.psconnect.com

First Printing, 2003

Printed and bound in Canada by
Friesens
Altona, Manitoba
Canada ROG 0B0

Cover Design CCCO NET INC.

Contents

Notice to Reader

The information in this book is for educational purposes only. Those who choose to treat themselves should consult with a medical professional for supervision. None of the contents of th book are intended to serve as medical advice, diagnosis, or treatment.

This book is intended to help people better understand the condition of psoriasis especially as it is misrepresented by mainstream medicine. In this regard, it speaks plainly. Althougl does contain information concerning successful methods used t resolve psoriasis, it should not be used as a method of self-diagnosis, since psoriasis is often confused with other disorders definitive diagnosis by a qualified medical professional is recommended.

Not all dietary regimens are suitable for everyone, thus any contemplated changes should be accompanied by a broader vie of your personal health status as determined by a physician.

Dear PCI Support,

When I first began the regime, I was diagnosed as being 88% covered. I was scheduled to begin a trial treatment, and opted to decline due to the unknown in the meds. I am pleased to tell you that I am now 90% clear, due to diet, supplements and your formula! I feel better than ever before. Some have said that it may just be in remission. That may be so, but I am enjoying no spots!

Thank you so much. You changed my life.

Janette (Texas, USA)
March, 2003

Introduction

"Men often stumble upon the truth, but pick themselves up, brush themselves off and carry on as if nothing had happened." – Sir Winston Churchill

Sometime around 1980, I noticed some funny looking, itchy areas on my skin. A dozen years later, full of frustration, I began the search for real answers. They came in ways I didn't expect. Those years were a long time to live in the dark - needlessly. In retrospect, I was let down by every doctor I ever saw about psoriasis, plus I could have paid for my children's university education with the money I paid out for useless medications. I became determined not to let this happen to others. My learned belief in the ultimate power of nature to heal has taken me down many roads in the search for the root cause of psoriasis, some of them blind alleys. Finally in the mid 1990's, the truth presented itself in a most serendipitous way in the person of Dr. John Pagano, a chiropractor in New Jersey. When as a professional bookseller I first read his book called 'Healing Psoriasis – the Natural Alternative', I knew I had struck the real source of the problem. The rest, as they say, is history.

Why this book and why now? There are two primary reasons. One, not much public attention is paid to the appalling way psoriasis is treated by the medical profession. Psoriasis is a lip-service disorder, as you have no doubt experienced firsthand yourself. Two, more voices need to be heard in a non-medical, almost political way, since it is the establishment that is keeping the truth about psoriasis from the public.

The result is this book.

The average person just wants to know what's wrong with them and what they can do about it. This book is about how things can change dramatically for you by incorporating some simple principles into your life – that is, if you adopt them.

viii

Chances are the average general practitioner is not going to appreciate this book, with some exceptions. Let me tell you why. First, a layman writes it. That's a disqualifier in medical eyes. Second, it refutes conventional statements about psoriasis. That's the second disqualifier. But there are other factors at play. One, you can't beat success. Two, after decades of battling medical myths, it's time someone said the things that are to follow, without fear of repercussions for career. And three, most importantly, too many people live in misery needlessly.

This book is not a wish list, it is based on the reality of information gathered over decades by medical practitioners, scientists, laymen, chiropractors, and countless others. To date the information contained herein has not been placed before the public to the extent that it should have been. If this book were a TV show, it might be 60 Minutes in the U.S., or W5 in Canada. However, it is not meant so much to be an exposure of medical shortcomings as it is an exposure of the real stuff behind healing. It is not meant to be as political as it is helpful. It certainly is not meant to be a medical text, a diagnostic tool, or medical advice. Rather, this book is meant to give you the truth about psoriasis and some healthy, natural dietary and lifestyle methods you can put to use. It will have accomplished its purpose if you conclude that you had better chart a different course.

Psoriasis is a complicated disorder, but this book is not complicated - intentionally. It is meant to be user friendly, with immediate practical application. It is a road map to the way out.

You hold in your hands the key to the so-called enigma of psoriasis. Yes, that's a bold statement, but one backed up with a history of success. Conventional wisdom teaches us that there is no known cause and no known cure for psoriasis, but you can forget about that now. There are proven, natural methods to heal psoriasis. Those who wait for the latest miracle drug to appear may not be interested. On the other hand, those willing to move outside of their comfort zone will find relief up to and including the complete disappearance of their psoriasis. Exploring solutions to your problem from every angle possible is very important. It is also assumed, and runs through the course of this work, that it takes mind, body and spirit together to be well. Your own knowledge of that may have to come later, once you achieve a degree of success.

No matter what your experience with psoriasis has been, your willingness to participate in your own disorder can and will make a significant difference in terms of a healing. This is not conjecture, but the real experience of many professionals trained in the field of natural medicine. Far from a fringe idea, the medical world is realizing that knowledge of self is a powerful force in healing. Psoriasis is a prime example of this principle.

If you have been unsuccessful in past attempts to cure, it's time for a new way. The discipline involved in a new effort is considerable and needs your daily attention, and just like any recipe, a missing ingredient can spell disappointment. Finding all the pieces of your personal puzzle is the goal.

We must face one fact. Since you have psoriasis, you are ill. Your system is out of balance, and until you re-balance it you will continue to struggle, no matter what you may be 'trying' next. Many people have achieved temporary success with various conventional treatments, only to have their hopes dashed when psoriasis returns, often worse than before.

A New View of Illness in General

A new view of illness suggests that no matter what illness you may have, there is only one disease called 'cellular malfunction'. Virtually everything that takes place in the body happens at the cellular level, whether it may be cancer, the common cold, or psoriasis. All disease has this commonality. With psoriasis, your cellular malfunction takes place mainly in your intestinal tract, as you will see. You may have other areas in your body that are malfunctioning as well, which can result in the 'domino effect', in other words, one problem leads to another, such as the psoriatic arthritis that develops in some people. However, when you methodically address all of your issues one by one, you can succeed in rebalancing your system. Since cell malfunction is the root of all illness, two possible causes exist - deficiency and toxicity. Most often it is both in combination that manifest the illness.

Rather than having 20,000 or so illnesses on the books, there is really only one – cell malfunction. If you accept that premise you are en route to your solution. Our current medical practices mainly deal with symptoms, as your experience with our medical system proves. Realize this, allow yourself the freedom to take a different approach, and you are on your way to a better life. Ignore this, and you are condemned to walk the treadmill of endless treatments.

This book is for the fed-up, the many people who know they *have* been on a treadmill and are willing to go all the way to put a stop to their illness. It is not for those who have an investment in their illnesses, who count on their psoriasis for focus in their lives. The changes required are not easy. They are natural and safe, though, and they will get the job done.

No one is being asked to accept this at face value. You must come to this place in your thinking of your own volition and experience. An earnest investigation of this book will shed new light on the whole range of factors that have been keeping you from the truth of healing potential. If you undertake this work, the strength of character that will emerge for you is going to be a godsend to your life. Aside from healing your psoriasis, the by-products of the work aside from psoriasis healing are a much-improved sense of well being, a zest for life, and a renewed optimism.

New ways of thinking suggest that diseases are *allowed* to exist in man. They are the end result of long-term abuse in the form of poor living habits, faulty nutrition, health-destroying environmental concerns and negative thinking. Disregarding the laws of nature in respect to environment, nutrition, physical and emotional needs leads to imbalance and disease.

Natural healing from days gone by was rediscovered in our time by the new pioneers in the field of health. It is a new science based on the inherent power of the living system to heal itself – a very old idea made new again after the gold rush of modern medicine failed, as indeed it has.

Man's body is endowed with an enormous capability to adapt itself to abnormal, adverse conditions. But this capacity is limited. When health-destroying conditions continue unchecked for prolonged periods of time, various disturbances in the functions of the organs and glands begin to manifest themselves. These may be in the form of fever, repeated colds and infections, enlarged liver, increased blood pressure, or as in your case, psoriasis. In most cases these are protective measures initiated by the organism in its effort to protect itself against the existing abnormal conditions. Ignored or suppressed by drugs, such symptoms may get progressively worse or change their nature and ultimately result in chronic pathological and degenerative changes.

It is becoming increasingly evident that today's medical approach, with drugs treating isolated symptoms, is unable to solve the problem of the catastrophic increase in degenerative diseases – cancer, cardiovascular disorders, arthritis, diabetes, AIDS, etc. The conventional approach of treating symptoms with specific drugs or other material remedies, without taking into consideration the patient's total condition of health and correcting the underlying causes of his ill health, is as unscientific as it is ineffective. A more fundamental approach takes man's environmental factors, nutritional patterns, and mental and emotional attitudes into consideration.

Treatment in natural healing is directed toward the elimination of the basic cause of the disease. It helps the body's own healing activity and restores the equilibrium and harmony in the function of the vital organs.

The practical philosophy throughout this book is based on the fundamental principle of intelligent cooperation with nature. Natural healing sees man as a part of nature, subject to its eternal laws. Thus, diseases can be cured only by the body's own inherent healing power.

The subject with regards to your psoriasis is cell health, specifically the cells of the intestinal lining.

The elements that make up a healing are:
1. Detoxification
2. Proper nutrition
3. Healing the intestinal tract
4. Balancing the immune system

Psoriasis, a disorder mentioned even in the Bible, has obviously been around for a long, long time. Lately, however, its incidence has been on the rise, and it affects virtually all age groups. Many things are said to play a role in the body's inability to correct itself – genetics, personal health history, body chemistry, and so on.

It will not be the purpose of this book to delve into the medical minutiae behind psoriasis. There is more than enough information about what is happening to your skin, namely that it replicates too fast in certain places. Scientists know exactly what is happening to your skin as it develops psoriasis. What they seem hesitant to admit is why.

One purpose of this book is to draw attention to the history of psoriasis as it relates to today's paradigm, leaving a large door of escape for you in the process. We have reached the point today where large organizations have been established to service the industry behind psoriasis. The average doctor doesn't understand any more about psoriasis than they read in their medical texts, the very books they consult when diagnosing it. These books all have the same basic information, which is that psoriasis has 'no known cause, no known cure'. It is the paradigm that our health industry operates with today, and doctors are far too busy making a living to challenge what they read in long-standing textbooks recognized by their profession. The result is that people are sent home with, at best, palliative treatments such as the creams, lotions and drugs that may have some temporary effect on the skin, but which have no lasting effect. Other more insidious treatments involve the use of methotrexate, a chemo drug that requires frequent liver biopsies due to potential destruction of this vital organ. Yet people willingly take this drug because it seems to work in the short run. And why wouldn't they? After all, a trained professional with a serious-looking license hanging on the wall recommended it to them.

This book aims to present an alternative view to the paradigm that exists in today's medical marketplace, and that's what it is - a marketplace. Practitioners can risk loss of career and reputation as well as license revocation if they make public statements against the prevailing views. There are no concerns of that type in this book. It is time to expose some little known truths about psoriasis for the public good.

People also tend to offer themselves up to medical professionals all too readily. Happily, there is a trend in Western medicine toward natural remedies, prevention, and holistic views of life. This will take time, however, and if you have psoriasis today, time is something you do not have. You would like to get your hands on a cure right now.

If this book is able to open your mind to the possibilities that exist for you and your psoriasis, it will have succeeded. The work will be up to you.

It can take decades for psoriasis to reach the surface, but it can take only a fraction of that time to rid you of it. Keep in mind that the day you first saw psoriatic lesions on your skin is not the first day you had it. Long before it first appeared, your body was fighting toxicity, and losing. The final result, not the first result, is the toxicity breaking out through your skin. It is astounding how we can be so sheltered from the reality behind psoriasis. Psoriasis is not the only condition that is misunderstood by many professionals. It is, however, one that can be fairly easily dismissed because it is not considered life threatening. But not being considered life threatening does not mean that it is not dangerous. Psoriasis has been associated, if not linked, to other problems; immune system deficiencies, arthritis, liver problems, and various digestive disorders. The fact that less than 500 people die each year from psoriasis complications puts it in the realm of 'harmless' to the medical community. This is admittedly a very small percentage, but when your doctor skims over the subject and throws a prescription at you, you begin to think twice.

Psoriasis is still controversial in terms of its origin, in spite of an abundance of evidence pointing to the source of the problem. People are completely frustrated by their condition, and by the confusing information they receive at a consultation. They leave their doctor's office asking themselves what they should do now, other than to go home and try to live with it. "They fly tourists into space now, can't they fix a simple skin condition?" The answer is yes, but the reason they have not done so is quite a bit more complex. Read on, and learn that the mysteries of this so-called enigma are no such thing. They are at best a careless attitude toward a seldom life-threatening disease, and at worst a blatant and successful effort to patronize and sometimes even exploit an often-desperate condition.

Thanks to Dr. John Pagano of New Jersey for paving the way for so many people. You should add his book, 'Healing Psoriasis – the Natural Alternative' to your arsenal. The one you have in your hands right now deals with the medical-system problem you have when visiting the doctor about your psoriasis. Once you understand why psoriasis is handled the way it is today, you will be ready to graduate to real healing. Otherwise, you will tend to accept what you hear at the typical doctor's office, and your pain will continue.

Read on, and find out why you have been living in a dark room with a light switch you haven't been told about.

Chapter One

Taking Charge of Your Own Case

"Examine your doctor, not the other way around."
- Author

"A physician is a person that treats a patient until they die, their money is all gone, or they are cured by nature." - Rene Descartes, 1596-1650

Spontaneous Healing,
A Reality Waiting to Happen

Dr. Andrew Weil wrote a book called *Spontaneous Healing, How to Discover and Enhance Your Body's Natural Ability to Maintain and Heal Itself.* In the book, Dr. Weil explains, "Motivated patients are a pleasure to work with. They are seeking information, which they will act on once they obtain it. Many of them have suffered physically, emotionally, or financially as a result of encounters with conventional medicine. Here are the complaints I hear most commonly".

"Doctors don't take time to listen to you or answer your questions."
"All they do is give you drugs; I don't want to take more drugs."
"They said there was nothing more they could do for me."
"They told me it would only get worse."
"They told me I would just have to live with it."

When it comes to health, we tend to take the easiest route if we can. We see the doctor; get some tests, maybe an MRI or CAT scan, prescriptions and even surgery. We place ourselves on the doctor's doorstep and say, "Fix me, doc!" We do almost anything to avoid our own participation, to convince ourselves that we are doing something about our problem, whereas in reality we're expecting THE DOCTOR to do something about it. After a while, we realize that it's not working. What's more, we too often discover that we are getting worse. Perhaps we'd get another doctor if they weren't in such

2

short supply. Better stick with the one we've got, even
though we now suspect that they really don't know what
they're doing. Now we know that if we're going to stop
this downward spiral, it falls upon us to do it ourselves.
A dawning awareness may also exist that the cause of
most of our health problems is what we're putting in our
mouths.

That 5-minute visit just doesn't cut it anymore. We're
not just disappointed, we're disgusted, and for sure
we're questioning whether we even like *ourselves*, much
less 'the system'. We're left with knowing that change
must come because it simply has to, or else.
Desperation sets in.

It gets worse. We're trusting the wrong people to take
care of us. According to an article in the Journal of the
American Medical Association, the United States placed
second last in a comparative study of 13 developed
countries. The subject? - Our conventional medical
system! The article went on to indicate that 20-30% of
all patients receive therapies that are contraindicated for
their condition, and medical errors kill tens of thousands
of people each year, making conventional health care
the #3 killer after heart disease and cancer. Stroke has
now moved to the #4 position. High-tech medicine may
be killing as many as 284,000 people per year,
according to JAMA.

Who should you trust then? Yourself and your intuition,
for starters. It's your body, and you should be the main
researcher. At this point, you may say, "But how can I
trust myself? – I don't know anything!" That's just the
point. You need a short education on the subject, after
which you can proceed to seek out 'consultants' to
advise you. Once you are done consulting with them,
you will be in a position to make an informed decision.
Always remember that doctors are not paid for curing,
they are paid for *treating*. There's a huge difference.

So here's the last resort - participation. It's your body.
The cells of your body are not functioning the way
nature intended, and it's time to do something about it.
Now picture yourself going in to see your doctor and
telling them the following:

"Look, Doc, my cells are all messed up, I'm full of toxins, I've got leaky gut syndrome, and something's got to give. You have to do something. I'm not getting the proper nutrition and my immune system is out of balance."

What do you suppose the response would be? This is *your* doctor, what do you think he or she would say?

Would it be -
"Gee, Bob, why didn't I think of that before? You need some serious counselling, and nutritional support. We're going to start you on a cleansing program right away and I'm going to refer you to a nutritionist, because I only had 6 hours of training in medical school on that subject. Then starting next week, we'll meet for an hour a week for some in-depth holistic work to get you started on a different way of life. We'll start by checking more than your pulse and blood pressure".

Or would it be -
"Gee, Bob, where did you get these ideas? Look, nothing you eat will make a difference to your psoriasis. What you need to realize is that psoriasis is a very stubborn condition. In fact you shouldn't be expecting it to go away, most people have it for life. It runs in families, you know. The best we can do is to stay with your prescription and hope that it helps. If it gets much worse, maybe we'll look at a course of chemotherapy, but don't worry, you don't have cancer."

Don't choose doctors who talk like this last one. Listen only to those who can help you make natural changes in your life. It's not the germs or genes that are the cause, it's the *terrain*. We don't 'get' sick; we allow sickness to flourish in our bodies. We quite literally invite it in by having an internal environment (terrain) that is conducive to growing the cells that make up the illness. We have arrived at a time in our society's health history when a powerful immune system coupled with prudent personal health management are not only advisable; they are the very essence of survival.

Let's spend a minute on the two main viewpoints of health and disease that have dominated our society.

Allopathic vs. Holistic

The Allopathic view sees diseases as external forces, meaning that the cause of disease comes from outside, then invades the body and the person gets "sick." This is the Germ Theory. The Allopathic view says that symptoms of disease or illness need to be dealt with immediately, usually by masking them or covering them up - suppressing them. When disease concentrates itself in the body, it must be isolated, then suppressed with drugs, burned out with chemotherapy, or surgically removed. That's the allopathic viewpoint, and likely the one your psoriasis has been treated with so far. Allopathy is a system of medicine that promotes the treatment of disease over the promoting of health. That's just the way it is seen by the doctors that graduate from the institutions that promote this kind of thinking, and that's all it is, a kind of thinking. Conveniently, it is part of an overall system dedicated to equipment, facilities, drugs and other tangibles that are put into place to 'treat' various illnesses. This is the system, and these are the tools. There is nothing more in this system. To find other ways, you have to leave the system, which is what is recommended in the case of psoriasis. Accepting the basic premise of this book that until the 'terrain' of your body is corrected you cannot expect positive permanent results means that 'treatment' is not what you are looking for.

The holistic view is the opposite. Holistic medicine says that the cause and cure of all diseases lies within the body. Naturopathic physicians recognize that true health is an optimal state wherein physical, mental, emotional and spiritual well-being are in balance. Some overzealous scientist types seemed to have run away with Louis Pasteur's germ theory and made a very distorted future for us all. Pasteur's theory, simply put, is that all disease can be traced to organisms that cause infection in the human body. Find the organism, deal with it, and the disease will go away. The holistic view is different. It maintains that by manipulating the internal environment to make it inhospitable for pathogens and infecting bacteria, disease cannot gain a foothold and does the only thing it can do, which is to fade away. Later on we'll learn that bacteria flourish in an acid environment, so it is certainly in our best interests to create an alkaline environment wherein most bacteria will die off – except for the ones that we call 'friendly bacteria', like lactobacillus acidophilus. Acidophilus aids in our digestive process and helps keep balance in our gut.

Let's now take examples of the treatment of psoriasis by both an allopathic doctor and a holistic one.

First, the allopathic doctor. They look at psoriasis as a symptom to be suppressed. The doctor examines your psoriasis and diagnoses it to be the common vulgaris or plaque variety. This is the scaly type that many people have. So there we have it, we have identified the enemy. Only this is not the enemy, this is merely the messenger from the enemy. The real enemy is in hiding, in this case deep in the gut. The doctor decides to shoot the messenger, and this is in fact what happens in most cases. There are many methods to shoot the messenger. Steroid creams are one. Light treatments are another. Drugs used for psoriasis dominate the treatment of this disorder and are not covered here because they are not the topic of this book, but there are many more coming, that's for sure. The newest one as of the writing of this book is Amavive, a T-cell suppressing drug that is sure to wreak havoc with a lot of people. Methotrexate, a chemo drug, is also on the rise in psoriasis treatment as well.

Whatever treatment the doctor deems best is likely to be the one used, and if it fails, another treatment will take its place until some level of success is reached. The false hope that proceeds from these treatments is costing psoriatics years of their lives and endless frustration for one simple reason – they are all temporary. Once everything has been tried, the pronouncement is usually made that you have a very stubborn case, resistant to treatment. This is a fancy way to say 'Hey, our stuff doesn't work.' Maybe you are relating to this. Maybe you've been down a long road leading nowhere and you are truly ready for something completely different, which is the holistic method of acting upon the real causes of psoriasis instead of the superficial one.

So the messenger has been shot by the doctor, or at least shot *at*. He might be wounded, but there are more messengers coming. They all have the same message – stop the process. Allopathic doctors see psoriasis as another symptom to be suppressed, another bacteria to be eradicated, except of course they do realize it's not a bacteria. It's a skin disease. According to them, presumably, it just 'comes'. It has no cause, or at least, the cause is 'unknown', as is the cure.

When the allopathic treatments have marginal or even reasonable success, the patient is declared 'in remission'. You are told that 'it will likely come back'. Sadly, the statistics do bear this out, but the fallacy is in the treatment. Of course it will come back if the treatments are temporary, or wrong-headed! The kind of pronouncements that people hear within the confines of their doctor's offices border on voodoo. On a more minor scale (or maybe not), they resemble the cancer pronouncements that still take place today that 'you only have 3 months to live'. How is this known? The fact is, it isn't known, it's part of the arrogance of a dehumanized medical system that relies more on statistics than on true human compassion. Many, many people have proved the predictions of their doctor to be 'dead' wrong, and they have gone on to live full, productive lives. Upon hearing of his patient recovering from a supposedly deadly cancer, the doctor matter-of-factly states that 'in certain cases, for reasons we don't know, the cancer simply vanishes'. That's just a more sophisticated way of saying 'Hey, I don't know, ya got me'. Well, the patient did prove them wrong, usually out of their own determination, and they avoided the medical hex as a result. Some doctors remind you of the person who once said, "I've only been wrong once in my life, I thought I made a mistake but I didn't". Doctors need to lighten up and be more honest with their patients, including their own shortcomings or lack of knowledge in whatever areas they are deficient.

The holistic practitioner, on the other hand, takes a 'wholly' different approach. Same condition, plaque psoriasis. Since the psoriasis is merely the outward manifestation of conditions in the body, let's start to rule out the possibilities and get to the core of the matter. This doctor knows from the mountain of material he has seen that psoriasis is an internal problem, stemming from leaky gut. Ah, but how did leaky gut happen? The doctor proceeds to check on a few things – Candida albicans, or yeast infection, for example. This destructive yeast infection, if allowed to flourish, can wipe out good bacteria causing an imbalance in the gut leading to permeable intestinal walls. A simple blood test can verify if this is the culprit, and if so, a strict dietary regimen can take care of it.

If this is not the root cause of this particular leaky gut, the physician can look further, examining the diet of the patient. Many foods contribute to leaky gut, and this will all be covered in detail later on. What we are trying to emphasize here is the process (holistic) that can be taken to discover the root problem and its beginnings. None of this requires drug intervention. Leaky gut is the problem leading to macromolecules and toxins entering the bloodstream. These are seen as 'foreign' and an autoimmune response is initiated. If the process is not stopped, that is, if the gut continues to leak, sometimes for years, a permanent autoimmune response is set up which can create other complications, diseases, allergies, and so on. It can become a cascade of problems for the patient, all dealt with as independent symptoms by the allopathic doctor. Not so the naturopathic physician, who sees the system as a whole. Tests for other pathogens can be made, eliminating them one by one until the real culprit comes forward. It may be Candida, it may be the nasty H. Pylori, or it may even be French fries. Yes, French fries. The destructive oils that enter the system from eating fries can act like acid on metal, destroying intestinal linings.

The naturopath knows that the internal workings of the body are so intricate and complex that no one person can grasp it at once, yet it must be considered as a whole. The body's sophistication includes the skeletal structure and the nerve complexes that branch out from it, the nervous system itself that modulates energy patterns and the flow of energy throughout the body, the various organs, the blood and lymph systems and the brain. Although these systems work without our conscious input, it is possible for us to intervene to a certain degree. Usually the body just goes about its business automatically, but if we are treating our body like a dumpsite, there are no fresh raw materials for the body to work with. Your immune system usually conquers disease without you knowing it. In fact, people carry cancer cells in them every day, but the immune system eliminates them. Change the terrain, and you set up the disease conditions of a more permanent nature. With psoriasis, the conditions are a poorly functioning digestive tract replete with toxins of various kinds, including parasites. Add a number of poor quality meals that sit in the tract for a few days putrefying and you have the terrain for 'leaky gut' to develop and perpetuate. If you allow this to continue, you have poor uptake of nutrients, further degrading your digestive strength and dissipating energy. You feel tired all the time, and this has an effect on every aspect of your life. Your work may suffer, your attitude may decline, and even your relationships can suffer. You need a new life with zest.

All of this takes place at the cellular level first, and then at some point the information enters your brain and you become aware of it. Make no mistake - this takes time, it doesn't happen overnight. Visible psoriasis is only the end result of a long process of deterioration. This is what you need to recognize and this is what you will need to address in order to rid yourself of it.

The inner workings of the body are one of the most phenomenally sophisticated mysteries in the known universe, so we shouldn't be arrogant in our approach to them yet many practitioners fall into this trap. The trouble is that it becomes *your* trap. A cursory or rubber stamp approach to psoriasis is not enough. A holistic approach is absolutely necessary because each of us is different. It is this uniqueness that is both a blessing and a challenge to healing of any kind. The life force that makes us up cannot be dealt with using technology alone. Surgery accomplishes its narrow mission, as does radiation, but balancing a whole human system is currently beyond the capacity of our machines.

The object of this chapter is not to take a run at doctors specifically, but to turn your head. You could say that conventionally trained doctors just don't know any better. In our society we look to doctors whenever we feel we are losing it, when we feel that we don't have control over our bodily functions or our daily well-being. Otherwise most of us keep away from them. After all, they are usually hard to get to see, and there is waiting time and so on. We do it when we need help, but after some period of time of doing this, we develop reliance on doctors to provide us with more or less instant remedies for what bothers us. These so-called remedies are all too often drugs, antibiotics and patchwork of some kind. If for some reason we are asked to make drastic changes in our habits, we may rebel. After all, we're looking for the quick fix so we can get back to whatever it was we were doing before we got sidetracked. This is the way it goes, and don't think it doesn't, because North Americans are the biggest drug users on planet earth.

In 2003, the CNN news network held a serious discussion as to whether every American should be on Prozac, the 'depression' drug, because it supposedly holds benefits for almost everybody. Aldous Huxley, the author of 'Brave New World' would say, "I told you so!" The point is that we are programmed for quick solutions, and doctors themselves are programmed the same way. They realize you want the quick solution and act accordingly, dispensing the 'best' prescription they can to put a stop to your problem. Most often this results in mere suppression of the symptoms. A simple example of this is in the fact that Americans spend over a billion dollars a year on antacids. It's a major industry. They do this because they get instant relief from the symptoms of what? – A badly functioning digestive system that resulted from poor eating habits. The same amount of money is spent on laxatives, for exactly the same reasons. It's madness.

With regard to your psoriasis, you should consider a doctor change if your doctor displays just *one* of these traits:

- Will not spend time with you on details
- Will not explain the condition, or doesn't understand it in the first place
- Utters the words 'no known cause, no known cure'
- Is not holistic in their methods of treatment
- Denies that diet plays any kind of role in your psoriasis
- Is not aware of a method for healing psoriasis
- Simply gets out a prescription pad

This is tough talk, but there's a reason behind it. In China, for example, if a person gets ill, they often take the step of firing their doctor. It's very interesting from a Western viewpoint. In China, a doctor's responsibility is to keep the patient healthy through advice, practical tips, and perhaps some herbal medicines as required. If this process goes wrong and the patient gets sick, they are within their rights to dismiss the doctor. When you stop to think about it, it's quite logical. In stark contrast to that, in Western society we usually go to the doctor only when we're already sick, so that he or she may treat the symptoms and not the cause. The symptoms go away if we're lucky, and we go away too, only to return when the next thing goes wrong. Many people are learning that this is not the best way to live, and that a little prevention goes a long way. It will be decades before this type of thinking goes 'mainstream' but some are not willing to wait for that day and are doing it now.

Let's see how The Great Myth acts out at the doctor's office. Take a moment and reflect on what you were thinking when you first went in with your psoriasis condition. Obviously you were looking for solutions, for answers as to what you should do, how you should behave, what you should eat, anything. Did you get them? Did you have a nice exchange with your doctor, whereby he or she collaborated with you and provided detailed information not only on your condition but also on how you arrived on the scene with it? Did you discuss lifestyle? Were you able to find out *anything* important that you could take out of the building and put into your life in order to relieve yourself of psoriasis? Likely not.

What you likely experienced was a slightly patronizing attitude 'explaining' that there is no known cause and no known cure for psoriasis, and that managing it 'as best you can' is the only way to deal with it. Oh, and by the way, here's a prescription for some cream. Chances are that this cream was a pharmaceutical. Were you told that there is possible long-term liver damage from using that cream? Were you told that the cream destroys layers of skin, thinning it out so badly that bleeding often results? Think back.

Now let's be clear about doctors, so it doesn't appear that it's just a case of doctor bashing here. Without a doubt some doctors deserve criticism in the end because something has to put an end to the loop tape that has been put into your head by the medical system. Here is what is on the tape:

"Doctors know what they're doing. They are highly educated and intelligent people who have years and years of training. If I don't listen to them, I can only blame myself."

Doctors are still people, but too many of us don't look at them that way. They see an M.D. That stands for Medical Deity. Doctors have lives just like us, they have children and go to their kids' games, they go fishing, they take vacations and yes, they have mortgages – sometimes big ones. That's why they have to get their practices cranked up, to keep the cash flowing like the rest of us do. And what's more, they resemble us in another important way – they make mistakes. Can we forgive them for that? In most cases we can. In some cases we can't. That's when we have to consider taking away their licences to practice. In one case, a surgical patient returned to her doctor complaining of pain in the abdomen, but was told that it was normal to expect a certain amount of pain after surgery to the abdomen. After several attempts to 'get to the bottom of it', she sought out another doctor who promptly ordered an Xray. What do you think they found? A fourteen-inch surgical tool embedded in her abdominal cavity that was left there by accident. Now that's got to hurt, and you can believe the doctor was hurting after the lawyer finished with him, or at least the doctor's insurance company was hurting. Doctors are usually immune from responsibility in this area, short of criminal behaviour.

In another case from 2002, both of a woman's breasts were removed because of a cancer diagnosis. Forty-eight hours after surgery the doctor came in to the hospital ward to present the news that the wrong chart was read and she in fact did not have cancer. Seven months after the surgery the hospital formally apologized, saying that procedures had been changed since the operation so that this 'type of thing' would not happen again. Interestingly, and certainly shockingly, the pathologist involved in the mistaken reading of the chart had not been disciplined to date, seven months after the operation. As disgustingly shabby as the hospital procedures were, it goes to show that even in dire circumstances as these were, doctors are not prepared to accept responsibility for wrongdoing. There are no Medical Deities, only people with higher degrees who make mistakes like the rest of us humans. We can forgive them for being human; for being arrogant and posturing, we cannot. Take your doctor's opinion 'under advisement'. He or she is a consultant only, not the final authority. That rests with you.

There's a thin line between taking a patient on and putting a patient on. In doctor situations, keep your wits about you and always ask more questions than you are asked. That way you will get what you came for which are answers. You didn't go to the doctor for questions. Too many people think they're in an interview session with the doctor, and that's because it's set up that way. Doctors need to control their time and therefore they need to control the 'interview'. Try controlling it yourself the next time you visit your doctor and you will soon find out how it works.

Essentially, you are contracting with the doctor for advice, whether or not you pay the bill directly or through some government program. You go to a lawyer for legal advice and you pay for it. The lawyer must provide some activity before you write the check. Doctors are a little different in the sense that money does not always change hands directly, which is unfortunate. If you had to slap $150 cash on the doctor's desk after the interview, things would change. You would have a tendency to be more demanding of the service, and you certainly would hold the doctor accountable for 'production'. As with a lawyer, if you are receiving shabby service, change to another with better service.

OK, so doctors are not perfect, and yours really does care about you, let's say. That is irrelevant when it comes to their fundamental knowledge about an admittedly complex condition, one that refers to specialists called dermatologists. M.D.'s take the path of least resistance (drugs) because they have to move on to the next patient. Other types of doctors, like naturopaths for instance, are often paid by the hour by choice and therefore have the time to properly research conditions and spend enough time with you to gain some practical knowledge of you. This leads to more specific application of remedy on an individual basis.

Dermatologists are another breed. Any honest one will admit that their practice is a cash cow. They can be both arrogant and abrupt. You see, *they've* got the cookie! You don't. You are a ticket to them, and they are so attached to the pharmaceutical industry that it should be investigated. They give you platitudes, tell you the same tired story as your M.D. did, and send you on your way with a piece of paper in your hand. Is any of this sounding familiar?

Fire them all if you need to, or if you would like to be more mild-mannered about it, just walk away. Keep them on hand for emergencies. Instead, get yourself a good naturopathic physician.

That's easy to say, right? You're scared. Your body is racked with psoriasis. If you desert the only person you know that may be able to help you – your doctor – then what will happen?

Don't worry, there is an answer; but first, let's talk about the politics of medicine.

'Mad Cash Cow Disease'

There is great relevance in learning something about organizations, particularly psoriasis organizations in your case, because in so learning you may see why a so-called cure has not been announced. It's analogous to the auto industry in a way. Does anyone really believe they have been unable to develop a gas-driven engine that gets, say, 100 miles to the gallon? Rumours circulated years ago that there was one, but they killed it. Pure economics. What would happen to the giant gas & oil industry if such an engine were developed? Whether or not it was developed, we are not likely to see it on the market; it simply does not serve the interests of those in control of that dominant market segment.

Let's apply this principle to a fictional psoriasis organization. You might even belong to such an organization, let's see if what follows applies to yours. We'll call our organization The National Association to Perpetuate Psoriasis, or NAPP for short.

Some well-meaning people who were interested in finding a cure for psoriasis started Napp many years ago. In fact, they had psoriasis themselves, so there was additional incentive to find a solution. The organization was set up as non-profit, as is fitting for a helpful group. A board of directors was established, and NAPP began producing volumes of information to share with 'victims' of psoriasis.

Time passed, and the founders passed away, their photos now adorning the walls of Head Office. Meanwhile, one hundred thousand members filled the databank. Additional staff had to be hired, and funding became a perennial and significant issue, overriding most other concerns. We're in a different ball game now. Annual membership fees were no longer adequate to float the organization, and 'other' sources of revenue had to be considered. One board member had a very bright idea, which brought in large chunks of cash without a lot of fuss. His idea was to request that each member include NAPP in his or her will. Thousands did, and with each 'passing', funds would flow in from probate.

Chapter 3 will deal with the other great source of revenue for NAPP, the pharmaceutical firms. These firms absolutely love a condition that doesn't go away. In fact, here's direct quote from one psoriasis organization:

"The research advances that will affect patients in the next 10 years will be largely funded by the pharmaceutical industry, and it's encouraging that they are now interested in this disease."

And why not, it's a condition that just won't go away, a convenient mystery, and one that will require endless treatment. In two words, Cash Cow.

So NAPP flourished, literature was disseminated to thousands of truly grateful people who were basically starved for information *due to the fact that their own doctors had little to offer in that regard.* You could learn more about the psoriasis condition from the extensive library at NAPP than you ever wished to know – about the *condition*, that is. About the solution, you could learn nothing. You could learn about the various 'treatments' that were offered in clinics and so on, but none of these were available directly from NAPP, because, you see, NAPP does not get directly involved in treatment, it is a research organization charged with finding a cure for psoriasis. Not only that, but NAPP does not endorse any particular treatment, it remains 'objective' in order to serve the needs of its membership better. Do you see how this works?

The purpose here is to awaken you to the realities behind the 'industry' of psoriasis. Are all of the people at NAPP part of a plot to take your money without consideration? Of course not. There are a great many good people in NAPP as there are in other organizations. This is not the issue; the issue is jobs. Imagine what would happen if a company came up with a sure-fire cure for psoriasis? Would NAPP fold? Not likely, but it sure would change drastically. People would run out and get that product, and cancel their memberships in NAPP. Downsizing would inevitably follow, and NAPP would be forced to reconsider their marketing (that's what it is - marketing) and perhaps take a truly information-only approach, a far cry from its present position of selling hope.

Reality Check #1

Doctors work hard. They have years and years of educational bills to pay. The average doctor is living to their economic capacity and needs a strong cash flow. They do not have the time to stop and analyse your entire lifestyle in order to 'work with you' on a condition that they may see as less than crucial, especially when compared to their *next* patient's problem. Besides, the book they consulted just an hour ago because they are not all that familiar with the intimate details of psoriasis, told them what to do - issue a pharmaceutical. Psoriasis organizations, on the other hand, are self-serving non-profit groups whose real purpose is to self-perpetuate, having come from noble beginnings. Some people who work in them have *never had psoriasis*. These organizations are fair game for 'Big Pharma', the pharmaceutical giants and the subject of Chapter 3.

Lack of research is not an adequate excuse for any doctor. Doctors who are people first will be happy to refer you elsewhere when they have hit the knowledge wall. The best you can do is to be your own researcher first but also find an informed doctor that you can hire as a medical consultant.

Chapter Two

The Great Paradigm Myth

"The problem with doctors is that they don't read
extensively outside of their own specialties"
- Dr. Russell Blaylock

"Beware the Barking Dogma"
- author

The view of psoriasis that is entrenched in the medical
jargon has both been accepted by the broadest range of
practitioners and methodically regurgitated. It is this:

"There is no known cause and no known cure for
psoriasis".

This is The Great Myth perpetrated upon the public, and
a seemingly petrified opinion based on nothing more
than historical repetition, both verbal and written. You
have no doubt heard the statement before, likely from
the lips of your own doctor. It also appears in almost
every medical document, article, journal and text in the
archives. Almost every one, but not all. You see, the
'accepted' view of most everything remains intact until
enough people move to another view so that the
remainder of people have no choice but to move over
too. This has gone on throughout history. Most major
discoveries and inventions have gone through a difficult
period of rejection before being accepted as reality.

The New Model for Healing

Our healthcare system is in the midst of a revolution.
Our old established models of how our bodies function
have undergone review in the last few decades and a
whole new interpretation has evolved, one that has not
been known to any great extent in the Western world.
Many medical practitioners, however, have moved over
to a new paradigm of thinking about the human body
and its workings.

A paradigm is considered to be the generally accepted model taken of a particular subject. Modern man has taken a "mechanistic" view of the human body until recently, when that view changed to that of quantum physics, a complicated field. The gap that existed between lab physics and, say, religious thought, has been narrowed considerably, and among the informed it has disappeared altogether. The Buddhist religion, for example, has long known that there are no borders in the universe, not between planetary systems, not between people, and not between the chair you are sitting in and the air surrounding it. There are only energy systems, constantly changing form at various rates. A cloud will change form very quickly, a block of lead won't. In the same way, you are changing constantly, and your interaction with your surroundings has a direct effect on your makeup. Energy in a concentrated form becomes something identifiable to us, and we give it a name. If you chop down a tree but don't remove it, it will become something else - soil. Its energy converts. So does yours. As humans, we have the ability to affect the changes we go through. An expression that is becoming well known goes "if you want to see what you'll look like 10 years from now, take a good look at what you're doing today." In other words, you become what you pay attention to. If it's Big Macs & fries, you'll look round in the middle and greasy.

We have quantum physics to thank for explaining in layman's terms a new way to see ourselves and the world around us. This will hopefully give us the insight to know that our actions determine our future. Our choices determine our future. As we choose to ignore our lifestyle transgressions 'only for today', then we have chosen to live with another day of psoriasis. That is the essence of the reluctance people have to embrace any course of action that doesn't have immediate results - we want to see results *now.* If they don't come now, we lose faith in their ever coming. On the other hand, if we demonstrate not just our willingness but also our courage to make better choices, we'll reap the rewards in our future life. Our *thoughts* become *things* - in this case, a better body. As you come to accept the wisdom of the view of the non-separateness of things, including your thoughts, you will see that you have incredible power within yourself, power that can heal. Many people know this to be factual. Seek them out, their books and their ideas. They will help you to arrive at this knowledge more comfortably.

What Came First, the Body or the Spirit?

A strong proponent of this new view of our physical presence on earth is Dr. Deepak Chopra, author of many fine books, and a leading authority on Ayurvedic medicine as practiced in the East. According to the new paradigm, we humans are not simply machines that learned to think through the process of evolution, rather we are spirits that created physical bodies. The physical body is therefore the product of all the ideas, beliefs and thoughts that one has had about it up to the present. To get your mind around this idea takes some doing, but if you read some of Dr. Chopra's work you will be able to do it. It is highly recommended, primarily because it can have a profound effect on the course of your healing. Once you understand that the human body is *transformed* continuously with your consent (active or passive), you are empowered to be involved in the process. *This is one of the central messages of this book.*

The quantum physics view of the human body relates to its ever-changing transformation. The body is not solid matter, but an energy 'field' that is subject to new perceptions. One of them is the perception of self-actualization. Put another way, *what you pay attention to grows*. Pay attention to your overall health and transform yourself into what you are - a healthy person without psoriasis!

To prove the point about transformation, here are some interesting facts:

- A completely new skin is grown every month.
- Every 5 days you have a new stomach lining.
- Your skeleton changes every six weeks.
- Your DNA at the atomic level changes every six weeks.

- 98% of the atoms in your body are replaced once a year.

The simple fact is that you are not the person you once were only a short time ago. Now imagine if you get involved in this process of transformation through your thought processes. What changes could come about? Is it really conceivable that your body was meant to have psoriasis? Hardly. It was meant to function perfectly, but something got in the way. Throughout this program we are going to work on those things. You need to reestablish balance in your body, whether physical, mental, or spiritual. If your present perception is that you've been 'attacked' by psoriasis, it's time to change it. The very act of changing your perception of the cause of your psoriasis will affect its outcome. Thoughts are real, as real as matter, and what you pay attention to will grow.

Let's take a simple example of a new level of involvement. Your stomach lining is new every 5 days, grown as new tissue from the elements in your body. Let's say that you have some stomach trouble in your life, perhaps an ulcer or chronic stomach upset. If you suddenly begin consuming only good fresh food, have exactly the right amount of nutrients that your body needs without any deficiencies, and are in peak physical condition with plenty of rest and a great psychological outlook, how long will it be before your stomach condition disappears? Five days? Ten days? A month? If you have a stomach condition, find out. Get involved in your own health.

It is important at this point to make a clear statement about the healing process - **you do not heal your body, it heals itself!** The only thing you can do is set the playing field up. If you provide the environment for your body to heal, it will do so. The so-called miracles of 'spontaneous healing' that we hear about are examples of people tapping into the universal intelligence that connects us all. Maxwell Maltz, author or Psycho-Cybernetics 2000, calls it 'Infundibulum', the opening of our beings to the funnel of knowledge that is universally available.

The Body/Mind connection is about realizing that we are indeed connected to everything; matter is only a concept, and is nothing more than a gathering of energy force fields which appear to us to be objects with their own separate identity. These are creations of our minds. When we finally realize that our connectedness gives us access to the universal intelligence, we are on to some truly powerful healing. Einstein believed in God.

How Change Comes About

It is well known that for a viewpoint to change, often the 'old school' must literally die off for the new generation's idea to become established.

In 1847, a Hungarian physician by the name of Dr. Ignas Semmelweis implemented the simple procedure of hand washing in chlorine to eliminate the germs that were causing a high death rate of women giving birth in hospitals. Instead of being hailed as a saviour, he was considered a heretic, and eventually he was drummed out of his profession. He died of insanity in 1865. The first man to discover germs died alone in a madhouse, literally scorned to death by his peers.

Nowadays, it would be considered madness not to believe the germ theory. It's funny how things change, but it certainly wasn't funny to the millions that died before the germ theory became 'popular'. In the same way, the current view of psoriasis is not funny to you at all.

At the moment, the paradigm is as stated by the medical profession. The problem is that the majority of people present themselves at the doctor's doorstep and accept as fact whatever their ears hear. The same can be said for TV news watchers, too many of whom do not understand that there is an agenda behind what they are hearing on TV, and it is not simply the reporting of facts. Witness the number of journalists who have lost their jobs due to lack of following the 'policies' of the company they represent. They are not towing the line.

Why, you might ask, would the medical profession put this myth forward in the first place? It's a good question, but let's answer it this way – it's just the way it is, it's the current view. At some point in the past, this myth was first proposed for lack of information. 'No known cause, no known cure' translated, means 'we don't understand it'. If you applied this thinking to the cancer industry, which you could, it would translate as 'there is no known cause or cure for cancer'. That would seem to be the case at present, but it doesn't explain why there is such a huge industry presumably searching madly for a cure. Why don't they just accept the statement 'no known cause, no known cure' for fact? The answer is – because the problem is too large. Not so with psoriasis. Only 3-4% of the population have psoriasis and they can live with it, according to typical advice handed out in the doctor's office. Most people with psoriasis would reply 'OK, buster, *you* try it!'

So the cancer industry strives to find the solution, the cure, because when they do, there will be even more money on the table than there is now. Soon one out of every two people will develop some form of cancer. Let's say that a special chemical derivative was discovered that was able to completely heal cancer. What do you suppose a treatment would cost? A hundred dollars? A thousand? How about a hundred thousand? We would suggest the latter. The point here is that when the problem is large enough, people will invest in a solution. As you will see later, a solution for psoriasis involves simplicity itself – detoxification, fortification of the intestines, and proper maintenance of the digestive tract – all relatively inexpensive. Compare that to the current situation - lotions, creams, light treatments, drugs, and an industry set up to provide ongoing treatments, not solutions, not self-managed programs with an end to them. The existence of a widely known regimen to heal psoriasis is not in the interests of the companies that make such products. This point cannot be overemphasized.

We can perhaps agree that psoriasis is indeed a stubborn condition – and the word 'condition' is used deliberately – that defies a single method for healing it. It is complex to be sure. Modern allopathic medicine operates as a 'track' to be followed in a scientific way. Diagnose the problem, find the source, and apply the remedy. This does not work with psoriasis because it is an admittedly complex condition requiring a multi-faceted approach, indeed a holistic one. This flies in the face of the allopathic method of medicine, and so it becomes an 'enigma' in the eyes of the medical profession. There is not enough time in a medical practice for a doctor to move in with someone, analyse his or her entire lifestyle, and make a holistic diagnosis leading to an integrated plan to achieve a healing. If you are wondering at this point about just what plan *is* functional, you may wish to glance at Chapter 12, but we recommend that you read the chapters in the order they appear so you will be able to grasp the entire concept that you are being presented.

Webster's defines a myth as follows:

'A traditional story of unknown authorship, ostensibly with a historical basis, but serving to usually explain some phenomenon of nature.'

- ✓ Traditional story
- ✓ Unknown authorship
- ✓ Ostensible historical basis
- ✓ Serving to explain some phenomenon

Three strikes and you're out, with one for good measure. The psoriasis enigma is medical myth, no more.

Synonyms for myth are: fable, fiction, legend, falsehood, and invention.

What were the doctors of yesterday to do with this psoriasis condition? They had no idea. As in the Bible, it was 'the itch that wouldn't go away'. Psoriasis wasn't the only enigma, and doctors had their credibility to uphold. After all, their work was surrounded by science, the ultimate source of knowledge. Proof was needed before any declarations could be made about anything. One wonders what they are saying now about the current use of 'laying on of hands' in modern hospitals. Surely this is mumbo-jumbo, they might say, yet too many results have been documented for it to be dismissed, so the laying on of hands has been taken on as an 'alternative' treatment.

The Phenomenon of Edgar Cayce

A native of Kentucky with a ninth grade education, Edgar Cayce accurately predicted two world wars, including the years they began and ended, the death of John F. Kennedy and hundreds of other recorded events. In his book "Edgar Cayce – the Sleeping Prophet", author Jess Stearn begins the book this way:
"It was like any other day for Edgar Cayce. He went to sleep by merely lying down and closing his eyes, and then he started to talk in his sleep. But when he awakened a half-hour or so later, he realized from the faces of those around him that he must have said something very extraordinary. And he had. In trance, on that hot, sultry day of August 1941, in the same voice that he would have prescribed an innocent herb for somebody with the sniffles, he had predicted the destruction of most of Los Angeles, San Francisco, and New York."

However you might feel about this kind of mysticism, it has been shown to be accurate.

Edgar Cayce predicted with 94% accuracy the illnesses of many people he had never met. Further, he didn't know about the diseases he 'diagnosed', often at great distances from the actual patient that he also didn't know. His statements on the cause of psoriasis have standing today, but not with conventional medicine. No sir, no self-respecting doctor is going to attach himself or herself to a now-deceased photographer who made trance-induced pronouncements on diseases. Or are they? In fact, certain doctors *have* attached themselves to these statements, and for good reason. Many practitioners have put into practice the principles behind the pronouncements and have had tremendous success. This success has not made it to the front pages, however, to the ultimate suffering of the millions of people who have not been 'privileged' to receive this information in any form whatever. Let's be clear about something. Edgar Cayce did not invent psoriasis healing. Chances are he didn't even understand it, he simply had the ability to trance-divine the information from a source. Who cares where the information came from? It has been proven valid, and when dealt with in a systematic way with holistic methods, people get healed.

The same applies to the psoriasis knowledge that has accumulated over the years, indeed over the decades. Cayce was very specific on psoriasis, as Stearn reports. In one section of his book, he describes the following:

"Repeatedly, Cayce stressed there was nothing incurable, provided one got to *the primary cause*. There was no point in treating symptoms. Psoriasis was one of the first things I looked for in the Cayce readings. I had stumbled through a thin file on the skin disorder, when somebody mentioned that a local osteopath had been treating psoriasis successfully from the dead psychic's readings. One reading was for a twenty-five-year-old woman, bothered with the disorder for years. Her mother, a naturopathic physician, had asked Cayce: "What is the cause of psoriasis? What remedies will cure it, or what kind of treatments will do the work? How long will it take until complete cure is effected?"

As usual in health readings, Cayce got quickly to the point, picking out conditions of a complex nature leading to incoordination in the eliminating system. "While there is thinning of the walls of the small intestines and there are poisons absorbed through the system that find expression in the attempt to eliminate through superficial circulation, we find that there are pressures also existing in the areas of the sixth, seventh dorsal that upset the coordination of circulation through the kidneys and liver. These contribute to the condition causing the abrasions which occur as red splotches or spots at times."

The mother enquired if psoriasis always had the same origin. No, Cayce replied, more often from lack of proper coordination in the eliminating systems. At times, the pressures may be in those areas disturbing the equilibrium between the heart and liver, or between heart and lungs. But it is always caused by a condition of lack of lymph circulation through alimentary canal and by absorption of such activities through the body."

In spite of the clarity given by Cayce, the patient failed to follow through with the treatment suggested. She went to two osteopaths who both made fun of it, so she quit. This was 1944, and not much has changed since then. Today's physicians still scoff at such suggestions to the detriment of their patients. Medical Deities (M.D.'s) can engage in dismissals with impunity.

As Stearn goes on to explain:
"Cayce had better luck with his second psoriasis patient, a woman, twenty-eight. The diagnosis was similar. *The conditions that exist through the thinning of the walls of the intestines allow the poisons to find expression in the lymph circulation, producing the irritation to and through the epidermis itself. Through the warm weather these show the tendency for greater activity in the perspiratory system, causing greater irritations.*"

Five months later there was a progress report on this woman.
"The psoriasis condition cleared up completely, except in places of scalp; there was some flare-up, when careless of diet."

Dr. Olis Wakefield, the osteopath who treated the woman, had this to say about Cayce and his suggestions:

"If something helps a patient, even if the treatment is not medically authenticated, I am for it. After all, my chief concern is helping people, not establishing the superiority of one concept of medicine over another."

Amen.

Before you start fumbling through the pages of this book looking for the actual detailed remedies, more is included in Chapter 12, so just keep going for now, because it is important that you follow the road to healing in its logical order.

A More Modern, but Similar View

'Digestive Wellness' is a book written by Elizabeth Lipski M.S., C.C.N. It is a terrific book that would benefit any psoriatic. Jeffrey Bland, PhD, writes in the forward "Digestive Wellness opens the door to a new chapter in nutritional science". The jacket provides the outline of the details inside that elaborate greatly on the reasons: "Not only is faulty digestion directly responsible for a large number of gastrointestinal and related disorders, it is indirectly responsible for a vast array of seemingly unrelated illnesses, including arthritis, chronic fatigue syndrome, eczema, fibromyalgia, food sensitivities, migraine headaches, psoriasis, and scleroderma."

Here is the essence of the problem that has dominated psoriasis treatment for decades. The myth still rules the medical profession, which as was indicated, is allopathic in nature. Anything else not generated by recognized medical authorities is dismissed out of hand. This leaves the average patient unconnected to the information in this book, for example. They are left with the 'normal' treatments recommended by their doctor – steroids, light treatments, drugs. This is a never-ending cycle, and one that the treatment industry really appreciates. Under this kind of supervision, psoriatics will never escape. It is a shame when you consider what would happen if individuals were empowered to take charge of their condition with the proper tools. Their doctors would never see them again, at least for psoriasis, and there would be more relief for a burdened medical system. Books like this one are intended to be a part of that relief.

Reality Check #2

People don't like to be ignorant, and will do or say almost anything to avoid appearing so. This includes doctors. Just like the germ theory took decades to establish, the natural healing of psoriasis will take time to accept. In the meantime, the methods are working, just as the washing of hands worked for Dr. Semmelweis in 1847. The bottom line is that the human body has the capability of healing *anything* if given the chance. There is not a condition known to man that someone has not proven that principle with, and that certainly includes psoriasis. Dr. John Pagano's success in healing psoriasis naturally is undeniable. Don't listen to the mutterings of people who use eloquent language to simply tell you that *they don't know*.

Chapter Three

Big Pharma

"Bamboozling the American public on the way to
massive profits only earns you a slap on the wrist."
- from an article by Arianna Huffington entitled 'Drug
Companies – Sell Hard, Sell Fast, and Count the Bodies
Later' for the book 'Everything You Know is Wrong – the
Disinformation Guide to Secrets & Lies'.

Big Pharma, the not-so-affectionate name for giant
pharmaceutical firms, is not a person like your doctor.
They are political and profit animals, thoroughbreds of
money, and they can be ruthless in their pursuit of it.
They rush drugs to market through lobbying, knowing in
advance that they will kill some people. There is a
special lobbyist on the steps of Congress for every single
drug of significance. Imagine getting up in the morning,
your only job being to lobby congressmen to pave the
way for your company's drug. That's what it's come to,
and the implications are frightening.

Before we delve into Big Pharma's connection to
psoriasis, let's clarify a few things. It must be said that
without drugs, many people would have departed this
earth by now, perhaps even you. They have a place, and
that place is crisis intervention. What is happening in the
marketplace, though, is quite another thing.

The little known, but soon-to-be-famous Codex
Alimentarius, exemplifies the long-range plan of the
pharmaceutical companies.

Background to Codex

The term 'Codex Alimentarius' means 'food code'. It has
been around since 1962 but now it's getting serious, and
the implications for all of us are dire. The Codex
Alimentarius Commission is a subsidiary of a
combination of the United Nations' Food and Agricultural
Organization and the World Health Organizations' Food
Standards Program. We will spend a little time here to
help you understand its relevance to your life and the

lives of all people who are interested in health freedom. The Codex is a good example to help explain how it is that the pharmaceutical firms have managed to worm their way in to almost every aspect of our lives. The name of the game is control.

Health supplements and natural products that you may choose to put into your body ought to be a matter of personal choice. The Codex aims to change that. In 1996, the Codex Committee on Nutrition and Foods for Special Dietary Uses met in Germany to consider a proposal that would result in new binding global trade rules for health supplements. It is no coincidence that the power base for multinational pharmaceutical corporations rests in Germany. The word 'binding' means that if Codex is implemented, the new rules will supersede national governments. This will leave effective control in the hands of the pharmaceutical firms who already operate effectively beyond the control of most government regulations.

What does all this mean? Under the proposal, all new dietary supplements would be banned unless they go through extensive Codex testing and approval. The monopolization of unpatentable botanicals is at stake. There is an international movement afoot intended to destroy health freedom in every country on earth, and decisions are being made at the boardroom tables of transnational corporations. Although a benign-looking organization, the Codex will have long-range implications in this way:

The Codex wants to limit potencies of all natural supplements to useless levels, leaving the right to produce and sell the higher potency versions in the hands of the drug companies and the pharmaceutical companies. These companies are principally in Germany and France and are connected to the big drug companies worldwide. In the process, the powers of the FDA and Canada's Health Protection Branch would be severely curtailed.

Ultimately, all of this represents nothing short of an attempt to create a borderless world run by dictatorial and powerful central banks and multinational corporations. Grabbing control of natural products and turning them into over-the-counter prescriptions will ensure not only control in the marketplace, but the ultimate reduction of potency combined with higher prices under monopoly. The feeding frenzy has already begun, with many German herbal product firms being bought up by drug companies.

According to Zoltan Rona, M.D., a specialist in preventive medicine:

"The Codex process is secretive, documentation is generally unavailable to the public, and there is little coverage in the media. If Codex Alimentarius has its way, then herbs, vitamins, minerals, homeopathic remedies, amino acids and other natural remedies you have taken for granted most of your life will be gone. The name of the game for Codex is to shift all remedies into the prescription category so that the medical monopoly and its bosses - the major pharmaceutical firms – can control them exclusively. The Codex proposals already exists as law in Norway and Germany where the entire health food industry has literally been taken over by the drug companies. In these countries, vitamin C above 200 mg. is illegal as is vitamin E above 45 IU, vitamin B1 over 2.4 mg and so on."

Once herbs and supplements become classified as drugs, it's all over. Unlike non-drug herbs, which by law cannot make any health claims, Codex would allow for product claims. With the drug companies In control of everything, you can only imagine where all of this is going.

How does this tie in to psoriasis? At present, Big Pharma controls the main supply of products that are used in psoriasis treatment. These are predominantly systemic prescription medications that fall into four categories:

1.   Cyclosporine (depresses immune system)
2.   Corticosteroids (steroids – potentially life
       threatening)
3.   Oral retinoids – a vitamin A derivative (liver
       function & cholesterol/triglyceride problems)
4.   Methotrexate – a chemotherapy drug

Whatever your doctor's favourite might be is the one that will be recommended to you. In spite of some temporary success, the vast majority of people eventually have reoccurrences, sometimes severe. You would be best advised to simply stay away from all of them.

Tremendous amounts of money are spent annually on these drugs of choice in psoriasis care. They could also be known collectively as 'consumables' because as you may have noticed, they go on and on. You are advised to keep on taking them even though you do not heal. There is nothing wrong with taking preventive consumables; in fact, this is an excellent idea, if it is a whole food supplement for example. Many people now believe that the time has passed when supplementation was a choice. It has become essential to good health. This subject is covered in more detail in the chapter on supplementation.

Because Big Pharma loves consumable drugs, and because they also know that you will be a customer for life unless something goes wrong (like healing), they have disincentives in place to finding a real and permanent solution to psoriasis. Actually, they're not really looking! Their job is to market drugs. To believe that they are helping you is to believe that your car dealer is there to make sure you get the best possible break on the price of your car. They are responsible only to their shareholders and although they have to 'wine and dine' the FDA, to them the FDA is the enemy, the last roadblock in the way of so-called progress.

It takes up to *$15 million dollars and 10 years* to get a drug to market. To Big Pharma, this is lost time, and they use a lot of their resources to circumvent regulations. At the moment, there is a huge controversy surrounding the latest TV ads touting drugs. What is happening is very interesting, if not disturbing. Surveys have found that up to 40% of the demand for new drugs at the doctors is coming from TV ads. This may not sound like a problem, but if you stop to think about it, this is marketing in its purest form. First we create a problem; then we create a drug for it. We place ads for it on TV using some very healthy-looking actors who explain how much better they feel because of using the drug. Have you noticed how many 'new' syndromes there are these days? Are we really deteriorating so quickly that we have new diseases every day? In one sense, yes we are. In another sense, much seems to be contrived in order to have people relate to the problem and then seek the solution that just happens to be a drug. In the simplest marketing terms – create the problem, and then provide the solution. It's an old story.

As far as psoriasis is concerned, Big Pharma would say, "You're going to need something while we're working on the real answers." That something, as you know, is a patented steroid, a light treatment, a chemo drug, or the various topical ointments that abound. The *real* answers are already here, but in the closed circuit system that you have been exposed to, your chances of hearing about them are poor.

An understanding of the mentality of the drug corporation is helpful to gain insight into the reason that ultimately you will not succeed on that path. Primarily it consists of knowing that they are addressing symptoms, not underlying causes. As such, it is an industry that will continue to flourish, especially when you consider that people are being 'educated' daily, mostly through the television, to think in a certain way about drugs. Keep in mind that these companies pay extraordinary amounts of money to the best creative marketing minds around, and they are masters at subliminal advertising. Not enough TV watchers even think about the fact that the actor on the ad, someone who has just recovered from a debilitating disease because of Miracle Drug 'X', is just that – an actor. They have probably never been sick with anything serious, much less the illness being described in the ad. Start paying attention to these actors and you will see the manipulation that you are being subjected to in the advertisements. The disclaimers at the end of the ads would be the stuff of comedy if the potential consequences of using them were not real.

If you are the type to take things at face value, you have a special challenge when it comes to the 'messages' we receive on a daily basis. Some studies show that we each receive up to 16,000 messages per day. Thank goodness our brains are programmed to filter out useless information, otherwise we would all go insane. Try to think objectively, not as the advertisers would have you think, which is something like the following:

'Gosh, these drug companies are a lifesaver. It's a good thing they're working night and day to discover new and innovative drugs to help us with our problems. Just imagine how much money they invest before even one new drug is on the market. What great people!'

If you buy into that kind of reasoning, you are on the slippery slope to pharmaceutical hell, and if you're over 50, you will likely end up with more than 12 medications in your medicine cabinet, which is the average number found in the cabinet of the North American over-50 adult. It makes you sit up and take notice, yet it is astounding to witness the number of people who take it all in stride. Some people are almost proud of the number of meds they *have to* take each day – sometimes 30 or 40 in number. People who work in the natural health field acknowledge that some folks have an investment in their illnesses, which is another way of saying that they can't imagine life without them. Worse, the investment includes the attention they receive by having their illness, by being able to talk constantly about it as if it were their favourite pet. You probably know some people like that. After a while, you start walking the other way to avoid them.

Drug companies will spend over three billion dollars a year to advertise their drugs to consumers. That is a lot of money. Compared to their returns, though, it is next to nothing.

This three billion dollar investment is targeted directly at consumers to further trick them into believing that a drug approach is the best solution for their health problems. Natural health advocates on the other hand don't have millions of dollars to combat this propaganda. The result is a $500 billion dollar expenditure by Americans on pharmaceuticals, driven largely by ads. The best defence against this invasion of our minds is to avoid watching ads altogether, which is easy to do thanks to that wonderful invention called the remote control. The smiling faces of rosy cheeked adults frolicking through grassy fields because they feel better on such-and-such a drug just doesn't cut it with a discerning mind. These actors bear no resemblance to the real, chronically wasted people suffering not only from their original afflictions, but also from the side effects of the many conflicting drugs they have been issued in the name of relief. It's a grand illusion perpetrated by the best and most expensive marketing minds in the country, and you are the target. You should opt out of the game. Do we really believe that we are benefiting from all of these drugs to the tune of half a trillion dollars?

Drug companies are sharp. They have managed through lobbyists to make it possible for them to market directly to consumers, mainly through television. Two thirds of doctor visits now result in a drug being prescribed, as TV drives people into their doctor's office demanding a prescription for the latest wonder drug. Spending for prescription drugs is the fastest-growing category of health care expenditures. Not only have physicians been programmed for pharmaceutical use as a front-line defence, so too have consumers, even to the point of being suspicious of anything that is not a drug. Such is the faith in this system that doctors are now the third leading cause of death in the United States due to over prescribing, misdiagnosis, and plain bad management.

The advent of the Internet has been a great step forward. People now have the ability to find reliable and relatively independent information that has to date been in the protective custody of the medical profession. This is producing results as people educate themselves before the medical examination, allowing them to ask intelligent questions of their practitioner at the examination.

Getting to the root cause of any illness is paramount. Psoriasis is no exception, and once you have done the research, part of which is this book, you will be sufficiently armed to proceed into the future with one goal in mind – to rid yourself once and for all of psoriasis – independent of other people's confusion, including that of your doctor.

The Tentacles of Big Pharma

Transnational companies have that name for a reason. They literally transcend national boundaries, and operate in a global environment that supersedes politics and governance. Their marketing strategies involve crossover products that produce problems for which they also have the solutions. Take pesticides, herbicides and industrial chemicals, for example. There is no question of the damage they do, although very little testing is done on their effects on the human system. This is partly politics, and partly because they are not used directly on humans; instead, they have a secondary effect. Interestingly, when problems in humans do arise, these same companies are standing there with the supposed solution in the form of prescription drugs, animal medicines, and a variety of medical products and technologies. They also hold patents on cancer treatments and devices, and a multitude of non-prescription so-called remedies. It's absurd, and most people are unaware of the insidious nature of crossover products. Taken to the extreme, it is entirely feasible that these corporate entities have a 'cradle to grave' strategy, as some suggest. Let us not lose sight of the fact that they are, in the beginning words of this chapter, thoroughbreds of money – profit animals.

The merging of giants is an indication of where things are going, namely to cross marketing and ultimately control over as many aspects of life as possible by individual corporations. As their fields of influence intertwine, they merge to create huge conglomerates capable of effecting social change. As sinister as this may sound, evidence abounds if only you keep your eyes open and read a few papers. You might ask what this has got to do with you. The short answer is that you are being led down the garden path straight into the agendas of these corporations – starting with your first visit to the doctor about your psoriasis.

Examples of Giants

- Monsanto
- Merck
- Aventis
- BASF
- Dow
- Bayer

Monsanto is a company owned by a firm called Pharmacia which was created by a merger of Pharmacia Upjohn with Monsanto Company. It employs roughly 60,000 people globally in 60 companies, and is the controversial company involved in GM (genetic modification) crop technology. Many farmers will testify that their generational family farms are now under the 'economic' control of Monsanto through contracts for the provision of GM seeds. While GM crops are ostensibly intended for things like pest control, the ultimate goal may indeed be people control. Farmers who quite innocently signed contracts years ago now find that they literally cannot afford to switch back to natural crops. They are trapped. In one lawsuit that smacks of Big Brother, Monsanto successfully sued a Saskatchewan farmer in Canada because his crops, which were non-GM, had been cross-pollinated in the wind by his neighbour's GM crop seeds. The settlement forced him to pay Monsanto for 'stealing' GM products. At last word, an appeal was launched – truly a David vs. Goliath scenario.

Thousands of toxic chemicals are also impregnated into products that we come in intimate contact with every day. These products generally have woefully inadequate testing. Synthetic chemicals are found in clothing, furniture, bedding, paper, food storage containers, building materials, pillow feathers, pillow covers, inks, mattresses, food, cosmetics, carbonless paper, fragrances, and tampons. A wide variety of fat-soluble pesticides are even impregnated into animal feed (fat soluble means it stores in fat). One of the reasons this is done is to cut down on flies in the barnyard. The fecal matter becomes so toxic that it ends up killing the flies! So the question is - does the animal fat cause us to get dosed with low levels of this stuff?

Most of the public is completely unaware of how pervasive toxic chemicals are in our homes and offices. If it were just one or two of the chemicals -- the effects might be tolerable. But that is not the case at all because the relentless cumulative and synergistic effects of these chemicals are causing great harm to human, animal and environmental health.

When we and our animals suffer from symptoms or become ill, or even have trouble with our reproductive systems, we spend many thousands of dollars on medical imaging, tests, treatments, operations, hospitals and drugs. This is a never-ending cycle of profit that is the envy of many other businesses. Again this year the chemical/pharmaceutical industry was declared the most profitable industry in the world. What a business to be in!

Altruism, or Mere Greed?

Subtle techniques are used to convince us that drug companies are altruistic. Although some front line workers in drug companies may have higher vision as humans, the real subject is a corporation. There's a huge difference. The companies themselves are certainly not altruistic. They are in the business of profit, of moving product, the more the merrier for the shareholders. Anything to prevent that process would be self-defeating, thus these companies support only efforts that lead people to their doorstep rather than in the opposite direction. This should be so obvious that it need not be mentioned; yet people continue to be taken in by the ads and the rhetoric. Don't be one of them. Educate yourself as quickly as you can.

Reality Check #3

Advertising works. Any sales person realizes that you must repeatedly contact someone, often as many as a dozen times, before you make a hit. Drug companies are among the best on the planet at this. Governments need them to keep things under control, so concessions are made. The only future a drug company has is if you take their products on a permanent basis. To accomplish their purpose, they will stop at almost nothing. Tobacco companies 'borrow' your body for a few decades until it is used up. Other types of drug companies convince you that life without them is just not worth living. No one is telling you any different.

40

Chapter Four

The Reality of Leaky Gut Syndrome

"There is no known cause and no known cure for psoriasis" - National Psoriasis Foundation

"Any new theory first is attacked as absurd, then admitted to be true, but obvious and insignificant. Finally it seems to be important; so important that its adversaries claim that they themselves discovered it." - William James

The Problem Area

The small intestine is the area of concern, coupled with proper care of the colon, which is discussed in the next chapter.

The flexed area between the duodenum and the jejunum in the small intestine is where the thinning of the intestinal walls takes place. Toxic leakage overloads the organs of elimination and the result is skin eruptions. Whether genetic in origin, or as a result of dietary/lifestyle habits, this problem can be dealt with by strengthening the walls of the small intestine, cleansing the colon, and improving dietary habits. This is the work you have ahead of you, but it can be done by anyone.

Leaky Gut Syndrome is not a new theory; it is established scientific fact. You can even order up a lab kit to find out if you have it. Leaky Gut is simply not treated as important (yet) in the treatment of psoriasis, and won't be until enough people step forward and take matters into their own hands. When a well-accepted theory is in motion, it has inertia. That explains the clinging on to the old medical paradigm found in reprinted medical books – 'no known cause, no known cure'. This paradigm suits many people and organizations that would not benefit by a logical explanation of the cause of psoriasis and the methodical procedure to be taken to heal it.

The Science Behind Leaky Gut Syndrome

We will be moving along to the supreme importance of digestive health in the next chapter, but for now let's explain the fundamentals of what is crudely but appropriately called Leaky Gut Syndrome, which we will refer to throughout this book as LGS.

In order to understand how LGS is at the root of your psoriasis problem, you need to understand the mechanics. The following chronic disorders have a commonality with LGS, in fact you may also be dealing with one or more of them in your life.

Irritable Bowel Syndrome
Spastic Colon
Crohn's Disease
Chronic Colitis
Regional Ileitis
Esophageal Reflux
Malabsorption Syndrome
Candida albicans

What your Digestive Tract is, and What it is Not

The digestive tract *is* a closed system from one end to the other. Actually, the intestinal tract is considered to be *outside* of the body. It contains not only the nutrients that allow for our survival, but also the toxic wastes that we have ingested in one form or another that would kill us if they entered the body all at once. The Chinese have a saying – 'Death by a thousand cuts'. You can be killed quickly, or slowly. When the 'closed' system leaks into the bloodstream, security has been broken and your castle is being stormed. Many people are dying a death by a thousand cuts, most of them unwittingly. We hope to change that by providing you with a full understanding of the importance of attending to your gut on a daily basis, and not only achieving resolution of your psoriasis, but learning the true meaning of 'optimal health' as well as having a wonderful new vigour.

Our Digestive Tracts Live Outside Us

Our digestive tracts work as a single unit from one end to the other, and they are considered a closed system. Nothing gets in except by the mouth, and waste is expelled at the other end.

From top to bottom, this unit is comprised of the:

Mouth
Throat
Esophagus
Stomach
Small intestine
Large intestine (colon)

What enters the mouth has to be broken down, yet everything will leave the body except for what enters the bloodstream, both good and bad. You might consider the digestive tract to be a giant filtering system. In the case of psoriasis, the filter is not working properly, allowing things into the bloodstream that don't belong there.

Let's explain.

When food is taken in, it is first chewed, although this process is usually neglected in our haste to finish the meal. It is suggested that food be chewed 25-35 times before swallowing, which has its reasons. First and foremost, the chewing of food releases the enzymes in the food, allowing for pre-digestion. When chewing doesn't take place, the stomach must do the breaking down of the food, which in turn can set up indigestion. The process is complicated, but the idea is not. Be conscious of chewing your food and you will find much improvement in digestion overall. The other good reason for chewing is to break the food down into small enough particles to allow for assimilation or absorption once the food passes from the stomach. Larger particles of food can create havoc later on in the digestive tract. Chewing is a very simple step that you can consciously take to make a significant improvement in your digestive health.

Once the food is chewed, it goes down the esophagus and ends up in the stomach. There the body's digestive juices break it down further, and it passes into the next section, the small intestine, which is over 20 feet long. The body supplies more enzymes to assist in digestion, and the nutrients are then ready to be absorbed directly into the body through finger like projections called microvilli that line the intestinal walls. These microvilli have an overall absorption area the size of a soccer field. The result of this enormous 'absorption' area is to permit small particles of food nutrients to pass through the intestinal wall into the bloodstream. A few hours of digesting like this, and the undigested food is passed along into the final section of the tract, the colon, which is about six feet long.

Before the food reaches the colon in the psoriasis patient, however, the trouble begins. Years of bad eating habits, destructive and toxic foods, speed eating, and a propensity for damage to the small intestine, allow for erosion of the intestinal walls to the point where food particles too large to be absorbed are nevertheless passed through the walls into the bloodstream where they are considered by the immune system to be foreign invaders. The minute passages between the microvilli have been widened, and what used to pass completely through the body *on the outside*, has now penetrated to the inside. This is the 'leaky' part of 'leaky gut'.

What Happens with Psoriasis

The delicate cells of the leak proof lining of the small intestine live only 3 days before they are replaced. Because the intestines are quite a hostile place due to toxins, strong acids, undigested food, and trillions of microorganisms, you can imagine how easily this one-cell thick environment can be disturbed.

Sticky belts called 'tight junctions' hold all the cells of the intestinal wall together, but when disturbed they can break up or detach, forming gaps between the cells. When this happens, larger undigested food particles slip through into the bloodstream and the lymph vessels, where they are recognized by the immune system as invaders. If this happens often enough, it is called 'increased intestinal permeability', or leaky gut. Disease conditions arise when organs of the body, particularly the liver, have to constantly deal with this debris, overstressing organs as well as the immune system that is trying to respond to the invasion. Psoriasis is but one result and in your case, the one you will have to deal with. Many psoriatics have multiple problems, including arthritis, another autoimmune disease. Undigested, or partially digested protein and carbohydrate molecules along with unwelcome microorganisms can circulate in the body for years, wreaking havoc in many different ways.

It may ring a bell for you to know that leaky gut often begins after accidents, critical illnesses, surgery, severe burns, or even sunburns.

The nutritional demands in the small intestine are high. This could be said to be the number one corrective action to take in healing a leaky gut.

Other contributing causes of leaky gut:
- Emotional stress
- Drug or antibiotic overuse
- Alcohol
- Parasites or infections
- Candida albicans (yeast) overgrowth
- High sugar intake
- Food allergies
- Fried & deep fried foods

Since a leaky gut can be brought on very quickly, even within a day or two, it can also be reversed quite rapidly if enough attention is paid to corrective action. As with most things in life, though, the repairs usually take longer than the original damage, as with a car accident.

When the balance of the food leaves the small intestine and passes into the colon, it can cause even more damage due to putrefaction. With a diet high in bad fats and excess protein, the colon diameter becomes smaller and smaller as impacted, putrid and fermenting food impacts on the colon walls. This in turn causes further blockage, often constipation, and certainly straining at stool. If you grimace at evacuation, it's time to sound the alarm bells. There is no age when straining is either expected or acceptable. Anything but comfort on evacuation can be considered a serious sign of obstruction.

The Journey of Your Food

Your closed circuit digestive tract *is not* a toxic waste dumpsite, yet this is exactly how too many people treat it, packing their colons with several meals that stay in them for days, weeks, or months.

The large intestine, also called the colon, is discussed in more detail in the next chapter, providing information on how to best respect and nurture the colon. It is noteworthy that today the incidence of colon cancer is dramatically on the rise, reaching a position of third place in cancers.

The whole process of converting food to nutrients is fascinating in the extreme, especially when you consider that the food sitting in your intestines is still on the outside of your body. At a certain stage of the digestion process, nutrients are taken up into the bloodstream, and this is where things can break down. The entire process of converting food to nutrients small enough to be absorbed into the body is no mean feat, but a highly orchestrated and timed event that can go wrong at many places and in many ways. That's why there are so many disorders and diseases associated with the digestive tract, which is also the home of the human immune system. Seventy percent of immune system complexes are produced in the gut.

Let's trace some food through your digestive tract.

The Mouth

We'll be health conscious and choose carrots, which we place in our mouth for chewing. We chose carrots because in raw form they come with their own enzymes to break the food down. Cooking them at high temperatures kills the enzymes, depleting your own supply. Later on we'll discuss processed foods and their destructive effect on digestion, but for now let's stick with healthy food. As with any 'live' food, enzymes begin to break down the carrot even before it moves on to the throat. This indicates the importance of proper chewing because the act of chewing ruptures the plant cells walls, releasing the enzymes, which begin to do their job. Hasty eating, and lack of chewing leaves many enzymes intact and unable to perform their task, which results in passing along too much of the digestive job to the small intestine, which under normal circumstances should be receiving more 'mulch' than 'lumps'.

If you eat 'dead' food, that is, food without enzymes intact, your pancreas must produce them in order for digestion to proceed. This digs into your whole life supply, the total amount of enzymes that your pancreas is able to produce before it becomes exhausted and gives in. You need to help, and there is more than one way you can do this. The best way is to eat foods that have enzymes, and eat them raw. Fresh, raw fruits and vegetables are the best way and you should be eating 5-9 servings every day. Only about 11% of the population manages to do this, leaving 89% with a deficiency. Another way to get enzymes is to find a good quality enzyme supplement that you can take before each meal which will help prevent enzyme depletion of your own limited resources.

It is an established fact that as we age, our body's production of enzymes decreases, leaving us in many instances with poor digestion, which in turn results in poor delivery of nutrients to our bloodstream, poor energy levels and poor resources with which to offset the natural degenerative processes taking place every day in the body. Enzymes can have a lot to do with length of life, but in the main they have more to do with *quality* of life, a subject dear to this book and to your condition of psoriasis.

The importance of enzymes cannot be overstated, in fact without them, our metabolic processes would halt and we would shortly die. Enzymes are catalytic substances that make life not only possible, but also continuous. They are instrumental in every chemical reaction that takes place in the body in our various organs, tissues and cells. When we ingest proteins, carbohydrates and fats, enzymes are involved in converting them to build our bodies. The uptake of precious vitamins and minerals also necessitate enzymes. Even though you may have eaten well (but cooked), without enzymes nothing will happen. In fact, enzyme deficiency speeds the progress of cancer, heart disease, arthritis, aging, and many other conditions.

So where do enzymes come from? First of all, our own bodies produce them. We are born with a finite production capability of enzymes, a kind of life potential. We can use them up quickly, or slowly. If it is slowly, they will last a lifetime. If quickly, we deplete our lifetime supply and can deplete our lives in the process, suffering from many degenerative diseases. Enzymes are produced primarily in the pancreas, a small organ weighing on average only about 85 grams.

There are four types of food enzymes:
1. Lipase – breaks down fat
2. Protease – breaks down proteins
3. Cellulase – helps break down cellulose
4. Amylase – breaks down starch

These enzymes digest our food by breaking it down into small enough particles to be able to pass through the minute pores of the small intestine into the bloodstream. The intestinal walls are lined with what are called 'microvilli', tiny waves of finger-like protrusions that increase the absorptive surface of the small intestine from its 22" length to about the size of a football field. This is an astounding feat of human physiology that stands in the middle of the road to better health. Disrespect it and we will suffer the consequences. The vast majority of people disrespect it every single day of their lives. They get away with it for a while, but not forever.

Let's move on from the mouth to the stomach.

The Stomach

The stomach receives the sometimes partially digested food from the mouth. Unlike the colon, the stomach does not have peristalsis (waves of activity that move food) as the colon does, but pushes or squeezes food along to the small intestine when the digestive juices are finished their part of the work. Food in the stomach is exposed to digestive juices that further break it down and turn it into real mulch. If digestive juices are inadequate or out of balance, we can suffer poor digestion, acid reflux, ulcers, or any number of disturbances. Proper food intake helps maintain balance in your system, including balanced acidic content. Whole books have been written on the subject of the stomach, but our purpose here is to track our food through the digestive system to the place where it and other factors set the stage for psoriasis.

The stomach consists of an upper (cardiac) section and a lower section. The upper section has no peristalsis, pepsin (protein enzymes), or acid, but holds the food awaiting a mixing with stomach acids in the lower section, further predigesting starches and preparing the launch into the small intestine, where nutrients will be taken up – or not!

The Small Intestine

Once introduced into the small intestine, nutrients begin to be absorbed through the microvilli into the bloodstream. This is exactly what is desired. The problem arises when large molecules of undigested sludge containing unwelcome large food particles and toxic materials are able to work their way through the same intestinal walls. How does this happen and why is this bad?

This happens because over time, sometimes over decades, the intestinal walls have deteriorated to the point where there is too much separation between the deteriorated microvilli, and these materials literally 'leak' through to the bloodstream. There they are recognized as foreign particles (undigested proteins, for example) as indeed they are. If this process continues, that is if the intestinal walls do not heal or recover, the problem exacerbates. The immune system comes to the rescue, sending antibodies to repel the 'invaders'. The result is an autoimmune reaction. This reaction can compound over the years, producing more and more deterioration in the digestive system, and allergies are often just one of the results.

So what causes this deterioration or 'thinning' of the intestinal wall of the small intestine?

Leaky Gut Syndrome – the Intestinal Lining

The small intestine is a bit of a paradox. It's job is both to let things pass through and to keep them out. It is a digestive organ as well as a barrier to toxins and macromolecules. The malfunction of this system can produce local results such as irritable bowel, or systemic ones like arthritis or joint inflammation.

When gut permeability is decreased, the result can be malnutrition, malabsorption, or even chronic wasting disease wherein the body simply fails to thrive. An increase in permeability, on the other hand, can play a major role in many clinical disorders like:

- Crohn's disease
- Allergies
- Celiac disease
- Rheumatoid arthritis
- Inflammatory bowel disease
- Psoriasis and other skin disorders
- Ankylosing Spondylitis

Repair of the lining of the gastrointestinal tract is fundamental to healing psoriasis. There is a special mucosal lining to the intestinal walls that is crucial to creating an environment for the efficient passing of nutrients, and nothing else, into the bloodstream. This lining is made up of, naturally, mucus. Intestinal mucosa can be negatively affected in many ways.

Contributors to Leaky Gut

Leaky gut is the end result of one or more of the following conditions that contribute to it. When you are looking for the cause of psoriasis, you need to look to

LGS. When looking for the cause of LGS, you need to use a checklist. One or more of the items below can contribute to or directly cause LGS. So as you can see, it's not simple to diagnose without a test. It's hard work for both the practitioner and the patient. That's just another reason you have to take charge and use a process of elimination to find *your* problems.

Checklist of Suspects in Leaky Gut Syndrome

- ☐ Parasitic infections
- ☐ Nutritional deficiencies
- ☐ Poor food choices (processed, fried, hydrogenated)
- ☐ Low digestive enzymes
- ☐ Low stomach acidity
- ☐ Alcohol abuse
- ☐ Highly refined and processed foods in your diet
- ☐ NSAIDS (non-steroidal anti-inflammatory drugs e.g. aspirin, ibuprofen)
- ☐ Antibiotics
- ☐ Steroids, including the creams you may be using
- ☐ Consumption of allergic foods
- ☐ HIV infection
- ☐ Intestinal infections
- ☐ Bacterial imbalance in the gut
- ☐ Aging
- ☐ Consumption of allergic foods
- ☐ Severe stress or trauma
- ☐ Chemical intake, starting with pesticides and herbicides
- ☐ Toxic intake

Can you recognize any of the causes of your own LGS in the above list?

Other Factors That Can Contribute

Air

If you think this subject is unimportant, consider the following. Since the Second World War, over 70,000 chemicals have been added to our society. A large percentage of these are unregulated, and many are expelled into the atmosphere in the form of industrial pollutants. We breathe these. Just keep in mind that if you can smell something, it is already in your lungs and has been assimilated into your bloodstream. Fortunately, our immune systems have the ability to recognize much of it and deal with it. If not, they will take up residence in our tissues and can wreak havoc. The other fact to consider is that in Chinese medicine, the lungs and intestines are linked in terms of energy flow. If lungs have problems, usually there is trouble in the intestines as well, and vice versa. You may have noticed this in your life already.

Avoid poor quality air whenever possible. One way is to consider a home air filtration system. These can be relatively inexpensive portable floor standing models, many nowadays with HEPA (fine particulate matter) filters built in.

Water

There's no avoiding it if you want to heal, and the healing abilities of water are discussed in Chapter 8 on rebuilding the body. Here we want to mention its toxic potential. In case you feel that water quality is not a very significant topic, let's discuss 'bad' water briefly.

A drop of water is virtually teeming with life, so it you're squeamish about such things, stay away from microscopes. The point is that water very easily turns into a dangerous, invisible enemy if not handled properly. That's why we rely on municipal water systems with chlorine and fluoride to deal with these matters. It's the lesser of the evils, yet for someone with psoriasis, these additives represent another form of assault on an already compromised system. Check with your local authorities to get a report on the quality of your community's water supply as compared to other communities. This report should list additives as well as percentages of harmful substances. If you are on a municipal water supply, there is not much you can do to change the 'system', but you can be aware. Once aware, you may be motivated to adapt your personal water supply to a better end product, as with filtering. Never use plastics to either drink water or store it. Research has shown that the plastics break down and enter the water, which means they enter your body. Plastics are made of some nasty material. With a little planning, you can avoid them altogether. Also, it's not the glass of water you drink; it's the gallons upon gallons that you put through your body, month in and month out, which can make a significant difference to your psoriasis. Remember, you have different needs than others. Take charge of your personal water supply.

Soil

Our soil conditions have a direct effect on our bodies. Modern farming methods involve huge volumes of chemicals, so much so that studies show an increase in breast cancers of women who merely *live* on a farm. When chemicals are added to mineral depleted soils, they kill off millions of life forms that populate the soil. Of course, the reason chemicals are added is largely to kill off the pests that can destroy crops. It's all economics, driven by the pharmaceutical firms through their agribusinesses. These firms make virtual slaves of many farmers who have been convinced to add the chemicals for various reasons, economic survival for their families being the primary one.

Aside from lacking nutrients to a large degree, the chemicals in soil are taken up directly into whatever food product is being grown, be that plant or animal. More chemicals are added in processing the crop, the final result being delivery of altered chemicals to your bloodstream, and therefore your organs. In case this disturbs you, there are many things you can do to avoid much of this - but not all. In today's world, total avoidance of chemicals is not likely, not if you're living in society. This is one of the reasons why careful supplementation is no longer a choice, but a necessity.

Chemicals in foods

As mentioned, there have been more than 70,000 chemicals introduced into our society since the end of World War II, many of them as by-products of industry. Cooking oil made from rapeseed is a good example. It was used as an industrial lubricant until some clever marketers discovered it could be sold as household cooking oil and voila! Most people think it is very good oil, but it's not.

No matter what combination from the list of suspects may be having an effect on your gut, think of your intestinal walls with their delicate microvilli trying to do the job of letting the good nutrients through to the bloodstream and keeping the unwanted out. Bacteria, fungus and parasites graze like cattle on the walls themselves, often with nothing to stop them. If your gut floras are completely out of balance, as with a bacterial or yeast infection, you have little chance to improve without taking remedial action. If you add antibiotics, you begin to kill off the good bacteria, adding insult to injury. The proliferation of antibiotic use has created huge problems of this type. These unwanted life forms will eventually consume you if you don't deal with them. The sad fact is that most people don't even know they exist until it's too late and they have a debilitating disease. Your intestinal walls are not the Hoover Dam; they are made from delicate material that is completely replaced every five days. Consistently negative influences on the walls result in inevitable damage, and if it is not stopped, it can produce LGS. This does not usually happen overnight, as many people believe. It can take years, even decades, before psoriasis 'erupts'. This may be likened to a volcano, which brews for a long time before we see the effects. Psoriasis is the final result of a long process of deterioration. Once you understand this, you can reverse the tide and begin on what is sometimes the long road back. On the other hand, because the body is so resilient, often the road back is a short one. It depends a lot on your general health, immune system, and attitude.

Entropy

Entropy is the process by which organization moves towards disorganization. For the human body, this means degeneration. The primary cause of degenerative processes in the body is deemed to be the *oxidative stress* caused by 'free radicals'. Free radicals are not people who used to protest on campuses in the 60's, but dangerous molecules that are missing an electron.

Free radicals result from many things:

- Oxygen
- Pollution
- Sunlight
- Stress
- Poor air conditions
- Chemicals
- Processed foods
- Excessive exercise
- Household products
- Electromagnetic radiation
- Hundreds of other sources in modern life

Actually, there is no escape, but there are things you can do to moderate your exposure to free radicals as well as counteracting their effects.

The only place that free radicals can find a replacement is to scavenge another molecule, in other words, a healthy one. When this process is multiplied in the millions, unchecked free radicals can be very destructive to the human body, affecting all systems including major organs, skin, and the body's ability to correct itself, even allowing for the proliferation of cancerous tissues. Free radicals are responsible for as many as 10 million oxidative 'hits' a day on your body. Fortunately, there is an answer, although most people still are unaware of it, and their doctors don't mention it because it falls in the natural realm. Free radicals can only be shut down by antioxidants. A major source of antioxidants is found in everyday fresh fruits and vegetables. If you kill the life in fruits and vegetables by cooking, boiling, or otherwise heating or processing them, not only are the majority of nutrients destroyed, but the antioxidant properties of them is severely curtailed. That's why fresh, raw fruits and vegetables are such a huge topic these days. It's only been in the last decade that we have discovered the phytochemicals in produce. Over 10,000 phytochemicals have been discovered so far, and we're still counting.

Parasites and pathogenic bacteria that reside in your intestines normally secrete their own brand of toxins, which have a damaging effect on not only your organs, but joints as well. In the process of destroying your mucosal lining, they send their toxins seeping through the intestinal wall into the bloodstream. Remember, they don't belong there, only micronutrients do, so now we have invaders. This is precisely what happens when these toxins and food allergens set up an autoimmune response. Arthritis is only one potential result.

Many people spend countless dollars repeating bowel cleanse programs over and over again, never suspecting that in spite of the fact that they are 'cleaner', they have not addressed their primary concern, the autointoxication presented by their leaky gut. In other words, they are wasting their time and money, and until they repair the gut lining, their problems will continue. Candida sufferers are a case in point.

So how do you know if you have leaky gut syndrome? There is a laboratory test you can take. Any naturopath can arrange for one and in the absence of that, the Great Smokies Diagnostic Laboratory in North Carolina can be contacted. They have a Kit you can purchase and return to their laboratory for diagnosis. This is best done through your doctor so that you have someone to consult with when the results are forwarded.

It's not whether you have LGS, it's how you got it.

If you're not up for a diagnostic test, then just go over the list, and tick them off one at a time until you have ruled out everything you suspect is not the cause of your leaky gut. However, if you want to prove to yourself that you have this condition, then get the test. It's quite definitive. You may have many other issues as well, but until this subject is dealt with, you could be skipping an obvious suspect.

Rather than the knowledge of leaky gut being a curse, it will be your salvation if you proceed on this course. You will not only escape from the clutches of Big Pharma, but you will gain back your freedom and your life will quite literally never be the same again.

This book is not a discussion about improving psoriasis; it's about resolving it. When this happens, the body will reach a state called homeostasis (balance). If you understand this, and are willing to apply the principles in this book, your problems may well be over. We'll get to the nuts and bolts shortly, but first let's begin with the source of your problem.

Conventional medical wisdom teaches us that there is no known cause and no known cure for psoriasis, but you can put that aside permanently now. For your own sake, please do. Those who constantly seek out the latest miracle drugs may continue to waste time doing so, but the fact that you are reading this right now is an indication of your willingness to explore another way. If you are willing to move outside of your comfort zone you will find not only relief from the symptoms of psoriasis, but its complete disappearance. You would indeed be an exceptional person if you did not ask the question at this point, "Is this REALLY true?" The answer is a resounding YES!

But why then are more people not healed?

LGS can be a stubborn condition. The following simple analogy may help to put the voyage to healing in perspective for you, and help explain a high failure rate. Let's say that you have a canoe and live on a vast river. The nearest port is 500 miles away. You fill your canoe with supplies and head out for the port. Will you arrive at your destination? The answer is obvious; if you keep paddling, you will get there. If you stop, you will not. Most people stop paddling somewhere between 1 and 500 miles. Others treat their mission as an epic voyage, and persevere to arrive at their destination, only to find that their lives have changed en route. It takes mind, body and spirit working together to achieve, which represent another type of balance. This explains why so many people fail to achieve their own epic voyage, in this case the voyage to healing. Conventional medicine is telling you that there is no port 500 miles away. This book is telling you to fill your canoe with supplies (knowledge) and start paddling. Your arms may be sore when you get there, but your life will have changed.

No matter what your experience with psoriasis has been, your willingness to participate in your own disorder can and will make a significant difference in terms of a healing. This is a crucial point, not conjecture, and represents the real experience of many professionals trained in the field of natural medicine. Nowadays, rather than being a fringe idea, the medical world is realizing that knowledge of self is a powerful force in healing, and psoriasis is certainly a case in point.

Reality Check #5

Is your digestion perfect? Do you have 'issues' in your digestive tract? How about bowel movements? Do you have more than one per day? If not, you have a problem. If you have used antibiotics to any appreciable degree in the past, you may have a problem. If you have had candida or yeast infection, you likely have a problem. Whatever your issues, you need to address them one at a time until they have been dispatched. Refer to the Checklist in this chapter. If you have been unsuccessful in past attempts to cure, it's time for a new way, don't you think? The definition of insanity is doing the same thing over and over again, expecting a different result. Finding all the pieces of your personal puzzle is the goal because one missing ingredient can spell disappointment.

Chapter Five

Digestive & Colon Health

"Indigestion is not caused by a Rolaids deficiency."
- Elizabeth Lipski, M.S., C.C.N., from 'Digestive Wellness'.

Old Story: You are what you eat.

New Story: You are what you absorb.

The importance of the colon in health cannot be overstated. It is central to the proper functioning of our entire system, as was recognized by the ancient physicians in Greece who agreed that 'death begins in the colon'. In your case, your new life begins in your colon.

Too many people either don't think about their colon health at all, or they have been accustomed to thinking that the colon and digestive system are nothing more than the body's dumpsite. Little regard is given to the profound interrelationship that the colon has to almost every function in the body. This will be further elaborated on in the chapter on our food chain.

The outright neglect of our colon health is exemplified by the disastrous rise of colon cancer in North America, which now resides as the number three cause of death in cancers. The story goes that when John Wayne was autopsied, they found a 40-pound mass in his intestines that was so impacted that you would need a chisel to break it up. This is neglect of the colon causing death, and a lesson learned a bit late.

Colon health is easy, but you have to know the basics first, and then you have to pay daily attention until you achieve a lifestyle – particularly a dietary lifestyle – that will automate the attention. The energy that a person experiences after a colon cleanse can be very dramatic, almost unbelievable in some cases. The biggest problem facing people is to understand the importance of colon health in the first place. Fortunately, you have that information in your hands now, plus there is a wealth of information from other sources.

The Goals in Colon Health for Psoriasis

1. Decrease the 'transit time' of food in the colon.
2. Eat to balance constipation vs. diarrhea, creating well-formed stools and ease of elimination.
3. Maximize high-quality nutrient intake to help heal cell walls in the small intestine.
4. Detoxify in every way possible.
5. Change bad habits.

Now, let's briefly deal with these one at a time.

Decreasing transit time

Food that is not absorbed is what we call waste. It contains indigestible material along with toxins, parasites, hormones, herbicides, pesticides and chemical residue from its manufacture. Why anyone would allow these things to remain in their body any longer than necessary is a mystery, especially when they have the power to change. When transit times are long, some of this nastiness is reabsorbed into the body, and re-circulates in the blood. To decrease transit time, increase fibre in your food, and eat natural foods like fruits & vegetables for example.

Eat to Balance Constipation vs. Diarrhea

Constipation occurs when the colon, usually due to slow transit times, absorbs excess moisture from waste material. Material from the small intestine arrives in liquid form, but if it has high mucus content, or is slimy, it moves more slowly than material with a high water content. This reinforces the importance of drinking a lot of water, making it available for this purpose. For someone with psoriasis, it is also crucial to eliminate all dairy products, considered to be the highest mucus-forming foods in our diets.

In the absence of water to help form stool, material is impacted, creating the 'lumpy' stool characteristic of constipation. Laxatives are definitely not the answer.

They most often irritate the colon further, and they have no cleansing effect on the colon whatsoever, leaving the older impacted material out of the process. Laxatives actually have no reason to exist, except for those who are unwilling to make the simplest changes to their diets, causing 'extra' bowel movements. Decrease transit times, and a feeling of well being is the result. People who take only the simple step of diet change have noticed dramatic health improvements.

Diarrhea on the other hand is most often the result of irritation in the colon. The body attempts to expel the irritation by emptying the colon often. Watery material has no time to be absorbed, leaving the stool in a mushy or runny state – the 'runs'. This is nature's way of eliminating unwanted parasites, or other material, so it's a good thing overall. Better yet is to clean up the environment and get back to balance in the colon. You do this with good dietary habits, clean unprocessed food, and conscious attention to our habits.

Maximize High-quality Nutrient Intake

Not only is it crucial for you to eat live foods, particularly fruits & vegetables, but for reasons indicated above, you need to allow your body to heal which it can only do with good raw materials. Given the scenario just outlined, imagine what years and years of abuse will do to the entire intestinal tract. It's no wonder psoriasis takes time to heal, but it certainly *will* heal if you set the stage. Complex carbohydrates coupled with smaller portions of protein, and lots of lubricants (water, primarily) will allow for the safe passage of food through the tract, leaving little behind. The leaving behind of waste has its own set of problems, principally an imbalance that perpetuates itself through neglect.

Consuming nutrients is not the same thing as absorbing them. It is entirely possible for quality nutrients to pass through your system undigested. The primary reason would be excess plaque build-up preventing absorption. Years of impacted plaque and mucus provide a virtual impenetrable barrier to nutrient absorption. That's why many people cannot understand why they don't feel better after starting on a natural diet. It can take a long time to clear the system of build-up unless steps are taken to deal with it before starting on a natural or whole food diet. One of the best ways to address a toxic colon is an intestinal cleansing program that can be purchased at a health food store or from a naturopathic physician. Make sure you get a reputable one with a history of success. Cleansing programs usually include a 'bulking agent' for expanding the colon, thus removing some or all of the built up plaque. Many people use these programs two or three times a year. They also include herbals that kill off parasites to rebalance life in the gut. Normally a person has about 400 species of bacteria in the gut. In sheer numbers, these life forms outnumber the number of cells in your body. It just makes sense to pay some attention to keeping them in check.

Detoxify in Every Way Possible

When coupled with undigested food, a toxic colon presents a challenge too great for your bacterial work force to deal with, leaving waste to build up on colon walls. This prevents proper absorption, and toxic materials that should have exited are now re-absorbed. It's double trouble.

Food that hangs around does so for three primary reasons. First, but not necessarily foremost, is that our bodies have become too acidic. A 7.4 pH balance is considered normal or neutral, and anything less is leaning to acidic. When this happens, our enzyme production goes down, leaving food either partially digested, or undigested.

This sets up plaque or mucus in the intestines which, when built up along the walls, prevents proper peristalsis, the lurching motion that moves our food along the tract. Simply put, you have moved from processing to storage. A severely distended gut is usually nothing more than several meals, even as many as ten, taking up semi-permanent residence in the body. That thought alone should prompt anyone to take steps to prevent that from happening.

The 'friendly' bacteria that we count on to reside in our gut have been disturbed, depleted, or killed off. These bacteria are essential to proper balance. When they are killed off, as with antibiotic use, other destructive bacteria are allowed to flourish, overpopulating the gut to the detriment of your digestion. The millions of friendly bacteria that live in the colon have the job of digesting the final remnants of food, leaving only the residue to be eliminated. You can have as much as three pounds of these bacteria in the colon. Without them, we would have no cleanup potential, so they really are our 'friends', the scavengers of our colon. The only method of re-populating them is to supplement, and to consume proper healthy foods. Probiotics (friendly bacteria) are therefore extremely important, as is the overall balance of them in the gut. Two common ones are Lactobacillus Acidophilus and Bifidum or Bifidobacteria, found in probiotic supplements at the health food store. Look for ones with a 4-5 billion count.

What Kills off Probiotics (Friendly Bacteria)

Antibiotics
Animal flesh containing antibiotics
Excess sugar
Antacids
Non-steroidal anti-inflammatory drugs (NSAIDs)
Prescription drugs
Soft drinks
Antihistamines
Fluoridated water
Coffee

An intestinal cleansing program is recommended, providing you have not had medical advice to the contrary for other reasons. Once you have a bowel cleanse under way, your body will commence to rid itself of toxic material. This does take time and often involves a period of feeling 'yukky' or out of sorts, but it is no more or less than the outcome of toxic material spilling into your bloodstream on its way to elimination. There can be a real flood of toxic waste at the beginning of cleansing, but shortly it abates and a sense of energy and well being usually follows, sometimes with a flourish.

Other easy ways of detoxifying are:

- Drink lots of good water
- Drink real lemon tea once or twice a day
- Take a milk thistle extract supplement for your liver
- Stay away from toxins, which includes processed foods with additives
- Get into skin brushing. Get a long handled natural bristle skin brush and brush your whole skin twice daily. This enervates your lymph system to flush out. It's the same principle as the Swedes whacking themselves with branches in their saunas. When brushing skin, always brush in the direction of your eliminations – up the arms, down the torso, up the legs, always towards the heart.

Changing Bad Habits

Habits are habits, good or bad. In the case of psoriasis, bad habits really hold you back. One man actually made the serious claim that he had to keep on smoking because every time he quit, even for a short period of time, his psoriasis flared up. While this may in fact have been true, his logic did not extend past his rationalization of his bad habit. He may have simply been 'stressing out' each time he quit, which could have brought on a flare-up. Or he could have been detoxifying, which is more likely. What he needed to do was face the reality of his bad habit and make the appropriate change to cure his psoriasis in the long run. He would have two positive results with the breaking of one bad habit.

Whatever habits you may have that you feel contribute to your ill health, take action. No one else can. Exercising is a habit, and so is not exercising. Eating before bedtime is also a habit, easily broken with a little determination (and some water before retiring).

Finally, get some help with the hard ones. You will be surprised how willing people are to help you achieve your goals once they see how sincere you are about making changes.

Reality Check #5

Do you have a 'waste dump' mentality about your colon? Is it a matter of 'out of sight, out of mind', or do you consciously examine your digestive health on a daily basis? Taking the Seven Day Food List Challenge as described in Chapter 10 would be a real eye-opener for you if you have a tendency to ignore your digestive tract. People whose front sides are bulging are ticking time bombs, and Mother Nature will see to it that you pay attention one way or another. Be pro-active.

Chapter Six

Acid/Alkaline Balance

"It is nothing less than amazing to see how quickly a patient responds, in a positive way, when the shift from acidity to alkalinity takes place." – Dr. John O.A. Pagano

The Alkalinity of the Body

This topic is crucial to your understanding of the psoriasis problem, and one of the most important in this book. It involves pH, the measure of the balance of acid and alkaline in your body.

When the body is too acidic, disease develops. For example, cancer cannot grow in an alkaline medium; neither can most bacteria, so as you can see, keeping the body in the proper ratio is mandatory for health. Bread is acidic, as are oranges. You would expect lemons to be acidic, but they're not, they have a strong alkaline effect on the body when ingested. You must learn not which foods are acidic, but which ones have an acidic effect on the body. There's a difference. A list of various foods and their relative acidity will follow.

The stomach lining has to be alkaline in order to counteract acidic digestive enzymes. Otherwise we'd burn holes in the stomach lining, which does occur in some people. All phases of digestion require a proper acid/base balance.

The ideal pH in the body is 7.4. The problem is, the fast foods that rule our society these days - hamburgers, fries, pop, pizza, and so many more, are acid forming. That means they lower the pH of the body; they are too acidic. When we eat them, our pH balance is disrupted. The many enzymes responsible for breaking down our food can't function and digestion is curtailed. The food just eaten sits there and literally rots. A sixteen-ounce pop has a pH around 2, which is extremely acidic. It would take about 50 litres of water to dilute this one pop enough to bring our pH back to normal. We don't do this, of course, so what happens next?

Since our blood must keep pH between 7.3 and 7.45 or we die, there is desperate work to be done. The body takes the extra acids into the tissues, muscles and joints to get it out of the blood, which becomes lactic acid build-up. As we literally pour more acid into our mouths, the body's only other desperate move is to 'make' crystals and salts out of the acid food, in this case, a pop. The result is the origin of uric acid crystals, the source of gout for one thing. Other crystalline problems are kidney stones, gallstones, and even cholesterol plaque.

We treat problems like gout with pharmaceuticals, yet the solution is simple – go alkaline in your diet, and stay alkaline. The ultimate problem, which can actually kill you, is acidosis, when the entire body becomes acidic in a disastrous domino effect of organ collapse and eventual death. Rather than look upon gout and kidney stones as 'conditions', we would be better advised to appreciate the body's ability to reduce our acid blood to these 'symptoms', saving us from certain death. This is an easy lesson that many people do not learn, and they continue to take a drug for a symptom rather than making simple changes in their diets to produce superior health without side effects. Just imagine what your internal environment is like after years and years of a continual acid-based diet! This is a war that has no end, except for the inevitable degeneration of the body's tissues, muscles, joints, bones, and all three trillion of your cells.

The Colon and Acid

An acid environment inhibits enzymatic activity in the stomach and small intestine. Recall that enzymes are the catalysts that break down food for eventual absorption through the intestinal walls and into the bloodstream. No absorption, no nutrients. No nutrients, no energy. No energy, no life. It's a simple equation. If you're not feeling 'up to par' or you long for your younger years when energy was something you took for granted, then examine your food habits. Most of us know an elderly person that we greatly admire for their unfailing energy and vigour. They amaze people with their zest for life, and outshine virtually everyone in their age group. If you know someone like this, they are undoubtedly an 'open' individual, so approach them and honestly ask them about their diet and lifestyle, and you will find that they follow a proper regimen. Rather than living a restrictive life, an 80-year-old like this will actually have more fun than a 40 year old who can hardly get out of bed in the morning. Moreover, the 40-year-old reaches for medications to get through the day, whereas the 80-year-old lived in a time before pharmaceuticals became part of our psyche, and thus by nature knows about personal attention to health. In the end, the real issue is not how long you live, but the quality of your daily life.

Let's get back to acid in the colon. By the time food gets to the colon, it should have been broken down and digested in the small intestine, but that hasn't happened in our example. The undigested food arrives in the colon where there are no digestive enzymes, so the food begins to putrefy or rot, precisely as it would at the garbage dump. What's worse, people who don't have regular bowel movements are really up against it, because this rotting food can remain in the colon for days on end. Some people are carrying around the last dozen meals they have eaten. They have virtually become a walking toxic waste site.

In this terribly inefficient process, brought about entirely by the individual's habits, there is another danger, that of poor mineral absorption. Trace minerals are crucial to our well being because they are necessary for enzymatic production, and of course they are delivered to us exclusively in our food supply. However, they can only be absorbed at a certain pH. By now you can likely see the chain reaction: an acidified body leading to decreased mineral absorption, reduction of enzymes, followed by rotting food. For psoriasis, this means slow (or fast) destruction of the intestinal walls by the toxic release from rotting food, creating a leaky gut. This sets up the autoimmune response in the system when substances and large molecules that have 'leaked' through large openings in the intestinal walls are recognized by the immune system as invaders. It's a vicious cycle, but one that you have total power to stop.

70

The following is a list of both acid and alkaline forming foods. It is self-explanatory. While it is one thing to read it and understand, you should take the additional step of referring to the list 'on the fly'. It will certainly help you to alkalinize your body over the months, and be of great assistance in the big picture. Maintain an 80% alkaline food intake to 20% acid as much as possible. It is the *ratio* that is important. Do not attempt to 'go 100% alkaline' simply because alkaline is good. It is the balance that is important, and acidic content is also necessary. Don't let all of this drive you crazy, just be aware of its relative importance.

Acid forming foods/substances 1 = high 4 = low	Alkaline forming foods/substances 1 = high 4 = low
Antibiotics 1	Apple 3
Aspartame 2	Almond 3
Cheese 2	Apple cider 3
Alcohol 3	Apricot 4
Almond oil 3	Avocado 4
Antihistamines 3	Baking soda 1
Amaranth 4	Burdock 1
Barley 1	Broccoli 2
Beef 1	Bell pepper 3
Brazil nuts 1	Blackberry 3
Balsalmic vinegar 3	Banana 4
Benzoate 3	Beet 4
Brown rice 4	Blueberry 4
Carob 1	Brussel sprout 4
Casein (milk protein) 2	Cantelope 2
Carrot 2	Chestnut 2
Chick peas 2	Cinnamon 2
Chicken 2	Citrus 2
Corn 2	Cauliflower 3
Cranberry 2	Cherry 3
Chard 3	Cod liver oil 3
Cow's milk 3	Collard greens 3
Canola oil 4	Chives 4
Coffee 4	Coconut oil 4
Cream 4	Currant 4
Curry 4	Endive 2
Dates 4	Eggplant 3

Eggs 4	Evening primrose oil 3
Fried foods 1	Fungi/mushroom 3
Farina/seminola 3	Garlic 2
Fava beans 4	Ginger root 2
Figs 4	Ginseng 3
Fish 4	Green tea 3
Green peas 2	Ghee (clarified butter) 4
Goat milk 3	Ginger tea 4
Goose 3	Grape 4
Gelatin 4	Hydrogenated oil 1
Goat cheese 4	Honeydew 2
Grape seed oil 4	Human milk 4
Guava 4	Kale 2
Hazelnut 1	Kohlrabi 2
Honey 4	Lentils 1
Ice cream 1	Loganberry 2
Jams & jellies 1	Lettuce 4
Kidney beans 4	Linseed oil 4
Lobster 1	Mango 2
Lard 2	Mineral water 2
Legumes 2	Molasses 2
Lamb 3	Mustard green 2
Lima beans 3	Nectarine 1
Malt 1	Nori 1
Maize 2	Onion 1
Millet 4	Olive 2
Monosodium glutamate 4	Oats 4
Nutmeg 2	Okra 4
Navy beans 3	Olive oil 4
Oat bran 2	Parsley 2
Pheasant 1	Parsnip 2
Palm kernel oil 2	Pepper 2
Peanuts 2	Papaya 3
Pecan 2	Peach 3
Pistachio 2	Pear 3
Pomegranate 2	Pineapple juice 3
Pork 2	Potato 3
Pinto beans 3	Pumpkin 3
Plums 3	Raspberry 1
Prunes 3	Rice syrup 3
Pickled fruit 4	Rutabaga 3
Pine nut 4	Raisin 4
Pineapple 4	Sweet potato/yam 1
Pumpkin seed oil 4	Sea salt 2

Processed cheese 1	Soy sauce 2
Rye 2	Spices 2
Rhubarb 4	Sake 3
Soybeans 1	Sesame seed oil 3
Sugar 1	Sprouts 3
Saccharin 2	Squash 4
Snow peas 2	Strawberry 4
Soy milk 2	Sulfite 4
Safflower oil 3	Table salt 1
Shell fish 3	Tangerine 1
Sesame oil 3	Turnip greens 4
Spinach 4	Wakame 1
String beans 4	Watermelon 1
Tapioca 3	Wild rice 4
Tofu 3	Sea vegetables in general 1
Tomato 3	Seeds
Turkey 3	
Vinegar 1	
Veal 2	
Vanilla 3	
Venison 4	
Walnut 1	
Wheat 3	
White beans 3	
White rice 3	
Yeast including alcohol 2	
Yogurt4	

Do your best, it will all help towards your goal of psoriasis-free.

Reality Check #6

Do you love your meat? Coffee? Pop? Other high acid items on the list? Can you substitute something else for that? What are you prepared to do to get psoriasis out of your life? The 'experts' will encourage you to get on with your life and live with psoriasis as best you can. That's not what is being said here. Make some crucial choices and get on with your life – WITHOUT psoriasis. Psoriasis healing is more about *choices* than anything.

Chapter Seven

Stress Factors In Healing

"The perfect no-stress environment is the grave."
- Greg Anderson, author of 'The 22 Non-negotiable Laws of Wellness'.

Attitude is Everything

Many medical authorities will attest to the need for the proper attitude in the healing process. If you do not believe this, then you should first do some research to conclude as so many others have, that this is in fact true. The main reason you need to do this Is that you cannot afford to have anything working against you that you could have as an ally instead. Henry Ford once said, "Whether you think you can or you can't - you are right." Wise words. Dr. Deepak Chopra, the author of many fine books, explains that a thought can be converted into a molecule, in other words your thoughts can become material reality. This is one basis of the current interest in 'imaging', the ability to project success on yourself through the thought process. So again, do some reading and enquiring. An excellent and fun book is **You Can't Afford the Luxury of a Negative Thought** by John-Roger & Peter McWilliams. This single book alone will likely set you on the right course if this is a problem area for you.

As you do your daily Progress Chart, give some real thought to the categories of emotional balance, relationships, ability to handle stress, and psychological state. Contrary to the belief of many people, a good lifestyle is not fast cars and opulent living. Rather, it is living within the person you really are, and being able to extend that person out to the world around you. Many people have not spent any time whatsoever in determining their true essence. However, some of those that have done so have made significant changes in their 'lifestyles'. It doesn't mean that you have to change careers, for example, but if you're an accountant by day and a musician in your heart, then you may want to look at altering your lifestyle to accommodate your musical talents, rather than abandoning your career as an accountant in order to starve as a musician (but don't tell that to Elton John). In short, take the time to listen to your heart, and make some small or even sometimes large decisions to go in the direction of your true self. They don't have to be earth shattering, but if you continue to watch TV while your woodworking skills are buried in the toolbox, you're missing a wonderful opportunity for peace of mind. Think about it, act on it, and take a few chances with yourself and others.

There is an expression meant to be humorous that goes something like "Stress is the urge to choke the living daylights out of some jerk that desperately need it." (expletives deleted). This is found on many desktops and office walls, and it is clearly a metaphor for pent-up frustration. Although many find it funny, the originator of this expression no doubt had difficulty handling stress, preferred to blame the rest of the world for his inner conflict, using humor to mask it. You do not have to be a 'mirror' for the world around you. If there are jerks out there, that's their problem - not yours. It simply means that you don't have to buy into it. Your true nature will allow you to look at these negative events objectively. Subjective viewers take everything into their being and try to absorb it. You may have heard the expression, "It's not what you're eating, it's what's eating you." Absorb only what's relevant for your personal well being.

Having empathy for a disadvantaged person, rather than being a downer, can be very uplifting when you consider that you have contributed to *betterment* in some way. Volunteers are among the happiest people around. A major best-selling book is one called "Random Acts of Kindness", primarily because it captured the imagination of those people who wished they could be involved in something like the reported incidents of daily life, in which strangers became involved in other people's plights, often changing their lives forever, anonymously in many cases. If you are looking for or feel you need some change in that direction, try a random act of kindness. It just could catch on, and become an important part of your daily life.

A Clinical View of Stress

A practicing psychologist with many years experience gives us an interpretation of stress as it may pertain to psoriasis. Here is what he has to say:

"Although psoriasis flare-ups often occur independently of stress factors, in general, most disease processes, including psoriasis, are helped by good stress management and a healthy lifestyle.

The reasons for this are obvious. The body has a very primitive reaction to threats to its safety. When the brain senses a threat, or there are serious demands to perform, the body responds as if it's actual survival is on the line. We call this Fight or Flight response. The body prepares for battle. We literally prepare to do battle or to run for our lives. Heart rate and breathing both increase, putting more blood and oxygen into the big muscles and away from the skin. We sweat to slip away from our enemies and to cool the fighting machine down. Digestion stops or dramatically slows down. Nourishment is not a priority since our life is on the line. Adrenaline and cortisone are secreted to give us energy and to reduce the inflammation of our expected injuries. Our mental focus goes away from our creativity and toward paranoia. We scan the environment for all possible threats. Even our vision can be affected. Our pupils dilate, making it possible to increase our peripheral vision and see our enemies attacking from the side, but blurring our central vision. Sex hormones are inhibited, as they are not needed in a "crisis." While all of these reactions are helpful if your enemy is a saber-toothed tiger, they are a liability if the stress is rush hour traffic or criticism from your boss.

The body can't distinguish well between actual physical danger and psychological stress and demands. Our bodies continue to respond as they have for thousands of years, except we have infinitely more demands, and limited opportunities to turn off the stress response. We are socialized not to respond with anger and fear in most situations. We "eat" the fear and anger. We don't punch the boss in the face and we don't run screaming out of his or her office. We don't usually slam our car into the "idiot" who cuts us off in traffic, although road rage is becoming more common. Panic Attacks, anxiety disorders, and depression are becoming more common as well, as our bodies and minds automatically respond as they always have, and we eventually have a failure of the amazing machine that we frequently abuse and neglect, our body. We must make it a point to turn off this response or else our bodies become exhausted and unable to heal themselves or respond to a real crisis. We need to return the body to rest and let it do the things that it has done in the non-computer/industrial past, the activities it was designed to do, at least part of the day.

Most stress reducing activities are simple and effective. Breathing is a good example. Concentrating on your breathing can be an effective meditation. Just empty your mind of everything as you focus on your breath. Try to breathe as infants do, allowing your belly to rise and fall. You can add other techniques, like imagining your lungs filling or emptying or exhaling while saying the word "relax" or "one" or whatever has significance to you. Decades ago, Herbert Benson, author of the "Relaxation Response" documented how effective meditation and breathing techniques produce the opposite of the stress response and produce the changes in brain and hormone activity that facilitate better mental and physical health. All forms of repetitive and focused activity have the potential of producing this response if the mind is quieted. Walking can be a good meditation if it is done with a Buddhist attitude of "When you walk, just walk." Meditations produce more than just a slow down of the stress response if done well. They can produce a healing response in the body. This is the most effective intervention and perhaps the most difficult. Damage control may be more realistic for most of us.

Again, most preventive and healthful activities are simple and common sense, but usually not followed with much dedication. Eating well, focusing on fresh fruit and vegetables, and avoiding non-nutrient "junk" food helps energy and promotes health. Learn to eat slowly and make mealtime a time to reconnect. Reducing or eliminating cigarettes, alcohol, and coffee is critical. Coffee in particular is underrated as a drug. One cup of coffee can double your resting adrenaline level. Exercise allows us to discharge our energy and use our bodies as they were intended. Lots of easy or moderate exercise is more healthful and consistent with how we evolved as animals. A good self-help book, like Peter McWilliam's "You Can't Afford the Luxury of a Negative Thought" can reduce the unnecessary worry that triggers the stress response. Spend some time in nature and away from overstimulating electronic devices. Take up yoga or Tai Chi. Call a good friend long distance. Turn the answering machine on. Read a novel. Get a massage. Spend some quality time with people who care about you. Go fishing. Play with your pet. Spend within your budget. Say "no" to that extra duty or activity. Even something exciting can be a drain if you are exhausted. Get enough sleep. Watch some comedies. Reactivate your spiritual life. Do less and enjoy what you do more. All common sense, right?

You probably already know what activities promote your health. Convince yourself you are important enough to pamper and nourish yourself mentally and physically, and you are likely to notice improvement in all aspects of your life, including your psoriasis."

Contributed by Don Scott, M.A., C.Psych.Assoc.

In addition to the accumulation of things you will be doing from now on, pay particular attention to your stress levels as they relate to the way you live your life. Perhaps you can pinpoint some changes that need to be made. See where you have been strong in your life, as well as where you need work. Try to incorporate needed changes into your habits.

Quieting the Barking Dogs

Volumes have been written about meditation so this will not be another one, but it is significant to bring the subject forward. Meditation is an ancient art and continues to this day because it contains truth. Not everyone is interested in meditation, but not everyone has psoriasis, and we are recommending that you find a method of meditation that is appropriate for yourself. It's not enough to relax, because even in a state of relaxation, the mind is chattering constantly. Meditation is meant to quiet the mind, to stop the incessant chatter. If you are not familiar with meditation, try this simple exercise:

- Sit in a quiet spot in your home where there are no distractions like TV, radio or people talking.
- As you breathe, draw your attention to your breathing and gently concentrate on it.
- Notice how your mind drifts away from your breathing and goes to a thought, sound or sensation.
- Bring your mind back to your breathing. Keep doing this until your mind doesn't drift anymore.

If you are not practiced at meditation, you will likely not succeed at this exercise on your first few attempts. It is amazing how much clutter is in the front of your mind on a moment-to-moment basis. The mind bounces around like a pinball, and you usually follow it. Once you master the art of meditating, you will find that thoughts dissipate and you are left with an 'empty mind'. The turmoil ends temporarily. Many people find that they are as refreshed at the end of this exercise as they are after a good night's sleep. Another comparison could be made to the feeling that you have outside after a heavy rainstorm. The reality of that situation is that the air is charged with negative ions, which give you an exuberant feeling. No matter how you come about getting that feeling, is it not worth it? No one is going to force you to meditate, but given the overwhelming evidence of its rejuvenating effects, why not incorporate it into your lifestyle? Ten or fifteen minutes twice a day can get the job done and the rewards are both physical and mental.

Facing a Backlog of Tension & Neglect

One of life's greatest remedies for stress is simple exercise. For those who are, shall we say, reluctant to make exercise a part of their daily life, there are some good reasons to take it up. They can be put in straightforward terms, so that your decision to exercise will be entirely yours, and you will not do it grudgingly.

First, let's compare life on planet earth long ago to what it is today.

The Primitive Life

- 24 hour days, sleeping sundown to sunrise
- Foraging for food - lots of walking
- Extended grooming and touching with other primates
- Fleeing or fighting in the face of physical threat

Modern Stress

- 30 hour days, intermittent sleep
- Processed non-nutrient foods
- Limited touching (often severely)
- Social pressures to avoid the "fight or flight" response
- Lack of physical activity

Plus...
- Noise pollution
- Pollution of water, air, food
- Chemical exposure - perfume, household products, soap
- Stimulating information systems like T.V., computers
- Demand to process excess information
- Light deprivation
- Sleep deprivation
- No afternoon naps and nighttime parenting
- Sleep disorders
- Media coverage of threats to environment, wars, T.V. violence
- People taking advantage of you
- Rising crime
- Concern for personal safety
- Physical health problems
- Children leaving home
- Job Stress
- Conflict with staff/supervisors

- Social contract effects
- Job security/insecurity
- Job boredom
- Lack of control over decisions affecting you
- Complaints of other staff
- Critical incident stress
- The weather
- Family incident & problems
- Alcohol or drug abuse in family
- Shift work of self, spouse, or children
- Separation or divorce
- Unresolved grief
- Elderly parents
- Children leaving home
- Children's activities/running a taxi service
- Marital or Sexual Problems
- Home renovations
- Resurfacing of childhood abuse
- Retirement
- Vacation
- Christmas
- Community Service
- Pressure by other to exercise, stop smoking
- Dieting/body image problems
- Fear of collapse of social safety net
- Panic attacks
- Negative perception habits (cynicism, pessimism)
- Personal tragedy
- Negative coping patterns (e.g. overeating, alcohol abuse, temper outbursts)
- Money problems
- Doing too much for others/putting others first
- The phone

All of the above, if considered together, would be enough to put anyone over the edge, but thankfully the human organism has developed some strategies to deal with things a piece at a time. I particularly like the expression I once saw on a fridge magnet – 'I try to take life one day at a time, but lately several days have attacked me at once.' Did you ever feel like that? We do have the ability, though, to effectively block out events, ideas, and troubles from our minds. This can work for or against us at times. Let's look at exercise as one means to block out our troubles for a period of time.

The focus we have when exercising gives us a breather, and the results can be substantial.

Exercise – the Wonderful Freedom

Psoriasis is caused by metabolic disorder, namely that of absorption in the intestines. Exercise changes the metabolism in many ways. The first is by increasing it, of course. The processes in the body speed up, blood circulates faster, and a cleansing process begins as a result. General stagnation is disrupted for once. Your sugar balance changes as more demand is placed on your body for energy. The lymph system moves. Deposited material in your flesh is circulated, including toxins that can be flushed out. Many people who have not exercised for years often begin too dramatically, and experience mild trauma as the toxic material that they have been carrying enters the blood stream in such amounts that their system is inundated and cannot handle its elimination. They literally feel sick, as if they had just been injected with a needle of toxic waste. It's sometimes called the 'healing crisis', and if you don't understand it, it can scare you off. Be aware of it.

So in the end, exercise is about elimination, circulation, rejuvenation, and when done moderately (e.g. brisk walking) it has nothing but positive effects for the psoriatic. The blood is carried to areas it has not been to before, and life at the cellular level is given a shot in the arm, so to speak.

Read a whole book on exercise if you wish, but this short explanation is meant to perhaps prompt you to at least go for a brisk walk routinely. Just try to incorporate some level of exercise into your daily routine.

Especially for Those Who Avoid Exercise

Some time has been spent in this book discussing our bodies' internal activity, especially at the cellular level. Our focus is not going to change during the short discussion here on exercise. Put as simply as possible,

the purpose of exercise is to enhance the transport of
oxygen and nutrients to the cells of the body. In
addition, it enhances the transport of carbon dioxide and
waste materials from the tissues of the body to the
blood and eventually to the organs of elimination, one of
which is your skin. Other than that, exercise could be
just a personal choice. But it isn't. Exercise is not an
option for those who wish a top quality of life up to the
point where they cease to be. Nor is it an option for
anyone wishing to detoxify. Movement is life.

The Benefits of Exercise as it Relates to Psoriasis

- Increased flexibility of muscles & joint motion.
  Especially true for anyone with psoriatic arthritis,
  but good for all.
- Helps draw away toxic material from these areas.
  Also good in cases of gout.
- Improves oxygen delivery throughout the body
  partly by enlarging arteries to the heart. This
  when coupled with good eating habits delivers
  more cleansing effect.
- Improves the way dietary fat is handled. Fat
  metabolism is particularly important to psoriatics.
- Improves immune function, leaving more fighting
  power for regular elimination.
- Reduces blood cholesterol and triglycerides,
  which means more efficiency in nutrient
  absorption.
- Helps in digestion and elimination.
- Release tension & anxiety thus improving mental
  outlook, self-esteem.
- Promotes relaxation and better sleep patterns,
  leaving the body refreshed.

The Effect of Exercise on Mood

Stressful life situations and the ability to handle them
can be greatly helped through exercise. Mood elevating
substances in the brain called endorphins, which have
been compared to morphine, are released with exercise.
The results are decreased feelings of anxiety, malaise,
restlessness, and depression. If that isn't appealing,
what is? Aside from all of the benefits for the general

population, psoriatics have every reason to incorporate exercise into their lifestyles. You don't have to become a long-distance runner to enjoy the immediate benefits of exercise. Walking is still ranked among the top exercises, as is swimming. Just do something!

Easy Steps to Get Going

- Recognize & admit the importance of exercise to your regimen for healing.
- Make sure what you are thinking of doing is OK - consult your doctor if your have special problems.
- Pick activities you *actually enjoy*. You may have to look around for new things. Try a few. Decide whether you're a 'loner' or would like to join a club or team of some kind. Group activities have more benefits than just physical, but if you like a brisk walk alone in the woods, go for it.
- Set times ahead for your exercise so that you won't have a built-in excuse not to do it, and do it often.
- Keep yourself motivated by varying your routine. Intentionally skip a session so you don't feel that you have your 'nose to the grindstone', but always return to it.

Reality Check #7

To admit stress in our lives is sometimes difficult, but everyone has it. Sometimes it's silent, and kills. Sometimes it just causes problems. Perhaps it's time to confront your own ideas of your stress levels, and the sources of your stress. They say that half of the solution to any problem is identifying the problem in the first place. Try it with stress, and see where it takes you.

Chapter Eight

Rebuilding the Body

"Question: I was under the impression that gut epithelium turned over every 4-5 days. Three months for intestinal permeability to heal seems like a long time when the offending agents have been removed. Could you comment on this?

Answer: Your question assumes that 'the offending agents' *have* been removed. Where is your evidence that we currently have enough knowledge to be able to do this? I suspect that at present our best endeavors may well be only addressing perhaps 10% of them. What we do thereby is to make a modest reduction in total load and as a result of nature being truly wonderful the result is that in spite of urban man's efforts in creating toxins many patients recovery processes are just enough to tip the balance in favor of healing. This would help to explain why the process is lengthy and why in some cases it is a failure. We can't yet be too smug about our achievements."
- Keith Eaton, M.D., United Kingdom.
From the book 'The Experts Speak – the Role of Nutrition in Medicine' 1996.

Let's Start with a Self-Quiz

How many out of 10 can you commit to?

1. I will make a deep personal commitment to myself to do this healing.
2. I will adopt this plan specifically to do so.
3. I will positively change the aspects of my diet necessary to succeed.
4. I anticipate a degree of control over my psoriasis by some of the measures to be taken.
5. I already do or will start to drink 6-8 glasses of *pure* water daily.
6. I will eliminate the nightshade plants from my diet starting now.

7. I will make the changes to prompt at least one regular bowel movement every day.
8. I will exercise at least 4 times a week for a minimum of an hour.
9. Carbonated drinks (sodas, *all*) have been eliminated from my diet.
10.   I understand that intestinal leakage (leaky gut syndrome) is the root cause of my psoriasis.

To consider yourself involved in real healing, you should have circled a minimum of 8. Anything less than 8 means that you may not yet be mentally prepared for the task. What's your score?

Getting yourself motivated is one of the keys to successful healing. The onus is entirely on *you*.

Let's deal with one of the subjects pertaining to psoriasis, namely that of fat, so we can move on to more important things. Theories do exist that psoriatics are unable to properly metabolize fat, compared to 'normal' people, so the subject may be more significant for you than for the average person.

It is not so much the simple consumption of fat that is at issue, it is eating too much of the wrong kinds of fat. This can seriously impair your healing abilities and may be a big mistake. High fat consumption can result in damage to arteries, cardiovascular problems, and restricted blood flow, which in turn reduce healing powers. For people with psoriasis, anything that inhibits the cleansing capabilities of the body is a threat to healing.

To reduce dietary fat, here are a few basics:
- Cut total fat by eliminating deep-fried foods, chips, avocados, and dairy products.
- Read labels of products you buy to determine fat content, and try to limit your fat intake to twenty to thirty percent of total calories.
- Cut back substantially on meat, including poultry, milk products, butter, margarine, and vegetable shortening.

- Eliminate polyunsaturated vegetable oils from your diet like corn, canola, peanut, safflower, sunflower and products made from them.
- Absolutely cut out trans-fatty acids from things like margarine and vegetable shortening, and watch for the words 'partially hydrogenated oils' on any food label. Walk away quickly from these items.

On the addition side, make essential fatty acids (essential oils) part of your diet as explained below.

Getting a Grip on Your Habits

We all have habits, in fact we couldn't live without them, but undoubtedly some of yours are damaging. Try this. 'Adjust out' one thing (at a time) that you know is not good for your system. It may be coffee. It could be pizza, sugar, alcohol, dessert, etc. That's perhaps manageable for you. And try to avoid a *deprivation mentality* when you do this. That's the main reason for the failure of diets in general. People convince themselves that their life would be happier if they were only able to consume what they used to, what they really would like to, and so on. In the same way that many ex-smokers can no longer imagine themselves smoking a cigarette under any circumstances, successful dieters have left the memory connection behind. This falls in the area of what is called neuro-associative conditioning, whereby your desires are directly linked to your memory of the last experience you had with the subject. A couple of experts in this field, and there are many, are Dr. Deepak Chopra, and Anthony Robbins, both of whom have written many hugely successful books. Look them up at your favorite bookstore.
So when you cut something out, do it with conviction and finality. When you're comfortable, adjust out something else. The time frame is up to you. Don't push too hard, but methodically schedule these events for maximum comfort while still doing it. Adjust out - then be proud of your accomplishment.

The Importance of Essential Fatty Acids (EFA's)

EFA's are essential fatty acids. Are you deficient in these key nutrients, and if so, what connection might they have to your psoriasis? As well as playing a critical role in normal physiology, EFA's are protect against heart disease, cancer, auto immune diseases, **many skin diseases,** and others. The commercial refinement of food containing fats and oils has effectively eliminated EFA's from our food chain. The results are deficiencies, allowing polyunsaturated oil products, for example, to contribute to heart disease, cancer and stroke without the offset of healthy EFA's. The essential fats, as found in flaxseed oil and fish oil for example, have shown to be effective in the treatment of many maladies such as eczema and psoriasis.

What EFA's do besides provide the body with energy:

Essential fatty acids regulate certain genes (over 100 so far) such as the ones that turn your fat storage mechanism on and off. That would seem to be significant, more so for some than for others. They also stabilize prostaglandin metabolism (hormone-like compounds made from EFA's), which affect linoleic acid levels. High levels of this acid can lead to allergies & inflammation plus these conditions:

- High cholesterol levels
- Prevention of strokes & heart attacks
- Angina
- High blood pressure
- Arthritis
- **Psoriasis and eczema**
- Cancer prevention & treatment

Should you take essential fatty acids as a daily supplement? It looks like you should. Organic, unrefined flaxseed oil is considered by many to be the answer to restoring the proper level of EFA's in your system. It is the richest source of Omega-3 fatty acids, which have beneficial effects on the above conditions, including inflammatory skin conditions. However, according to Dr.

Udo Erasmus, a world authority on fats & oils, Omega 3 oil by itself is not the best way to get the job done. You need a combination of Omega 3 and 6 oils. The proper ratio according to Dr. Erasmus is twice the amount of Omega 3 to Omega 6, which he has formulated into an EFA product (See Resource section). Check with your doctor if you're concerned at all.

To learn more about this subject, look for Dr. Erasmus' excellent reference book 'Fats that Heal, Fats that Kill' which is considered by many to be the bible on the subject.

Lecithin - You can live without it, but why would you want to?

Inexpensive and available in most health food stores in granular form, lecithin is composed of glycerol, two fatty acids and a phosphatidic acid. This combination can be useful in reducing cholesterol for one thing. By reducing serum lipid (fat) levels in the blood, cardiovascular risk is reduced. Lecithin has been indicated as a fat emulsifier, which means it can render fat more soluble, allowing it to be purged from your veins. That means a cleaner vascular system, better blood flow, better nutrient absorption and less risk for other diseases while you're working on healing your psoriasis. That's the primary reason it's recommended as part of a healing regimen. Unless you have a reason not to do it, put lecithin into your daily routine. The kind you'll find at the health food store usually comes from soy. It's quite palatable when mixed with orange juice, for example, but it can also be sprinkled on your food, or mixed in. Experiment until you find the way that pleases you.

Sugar - Your Mortal Enemy

Oh, no! Not more about sugar!
Can't we just forget it? I only have a little every week. What's the big deal?

This isn't just about sugar. It's about psoriasis. Sugar would merit a separate chapter in any health book, but there are already dozens of great books written on the subject. We do need to address the topic here in any case, because it is relevant in the extreme.

Here is an astonishing fact. Back in the 1800's in North America, the average person consumed the equivalent of about 5 pounds of sugar per year. Today, it's more than 150 pounds - *per person!* What's going on here?

What's going on is an epidemic. Type 2 Diabetes or adult onset diabetes is considered to be at epidemic proportions, causing all kinds of grief. What is different from the 1800's is **hidden ingredients**. You no longer have a choice - you must arm yourself with information as a shopper. Sugar has many disguises and it is very difficult to avoid. Even most people who avoid sugar get more sugar on a daily basis than is healthy, so if you're not one of them, imagine what you're getting. If you want to see how sugar is 'prettied up' in our society, check the website sugar.org, the website of the U.S. Sugar Association.

One of sugar's insidious effects is to strip away other nutrients from your body. Calcium is a good example. With today's concern for calcium loss, why would anyone consume sugar? The answer is simple - marketing. Once you become aware of the manufacturer's inclination to include sugar in almost everything made, you will see what kind of challenge we are facing. What you are missing when you get your calories from sugar is the nutrition you get from other foods you're *not* eating, so when people say they are addicted to chocolate and sweets, they're not far from the truth. Some sugar mixtures are linked to endorphins made by the body that act as opiates. No wonder there's binge eating and yo-yo dieting.

The Sugar/Psoriasis Connection

One problem with sugar and psoriasis has to do with fermentation. Fermentation in the gut can cause deterioration of the intestinal walls as well as re-toxification of material that would normally exit the body but is now reabsorbed. Gas is often a by-product. You are trying to strengthen the intestinal walls, not destroy them. The next time you experience gas, as everyone does from time to time, reflect on what you ate that may have set it up. The next time you can avoid it.

If you get a large part of your calories from added sugar, you won't get the good things like fruits, vegetables, whole grains, fiber, and the vitamins & minerals that whole food brings you. This is absolutely crucial to your well-being and particularly to the chances of healing your psoriasis, but just keep in mind that healing psoriasis is really not chance at all, but procedure.

Soda Pop – Cancer in a Can

Get rid of this. Here's why. A can of pop or soda can contain as much as 15 teaspoons of sugar. Try eating 15 teaspoons of sugar off the spoon and you'll likely be ill, yet nicely hidden in the can of pop, it tastes pretty good. Either way, it's deadly over time and dynamite for your psoriasis. Unwanted bacteria in the gut feed on sugar. There is no end of fluids to drink on the planet, and there are no excuses for drinking pop, except for the ones you make up.

The Sneak Attack of Aspartame

Aspartame is dangerous. You will notice many people who are weight conscious drinking pop with aspartame in an effort not to consume sugar. Little do they know that aspartame can actually *cause* weight gain in the body. This is as a result of the body being tricked into thinking that there is a shortage of sugar, and the body attempts to store up for the future.

The short story of aspartame is as follows. Because aspartame is classified as a food additive, the law does not monitor its continued safety. Once listed on a prospective list of biochemical warfare weapons by the Pentagon, it now is marketed as a sweetener in over 1,200 food products. In the body, it breaks down into amino acids and methanol, which results in formaldehyde. This methanol byproduct could be considered toxic if its content in aspartame is 1000 times greater than most foods under regulatory control. Is this enough for you to discontinue its use? If not, *this* might be. Aspartame, an excitotoxin, has been shown in animal studies to alter brain chemicals affecting behavior, and high doses of it have been linked to a craving for carbohydrates.

How aspartame breaks down

Methanol, from aspartame, is released in the small intestine when the methyl group of aspartame encounters the enzyme chymotrypsin. Free methanol begins to form in liquid aspartame-containing products at temperatures above 86 degrees F - also within the human body. The methanol is then converted to formaldehyde. The formaldehyde converts to formic acid (ant sting poison). Formic acid is a component of products used to strip urethane off furniture. Imagine what it does to your insides! Phenylalanine and aspartic acid, which comprise 90% of aspartame, are amino acids. When unaccompanied by other amino acids we use, however, they are neurotoxic. That is why a warning for phenylketonurics is found on EQUAL and other aspartame products.

In other words aspartame converts to dangerous byproducts, and nothing counterbalances them.

The American Cancer Society studied 80,000 women over 6 years and found that "among women users who gained weight, artificial sweetener users gained more than those who didn't use the products". What?? Have we been duped? Yes. And in 1991, the National Institutes of Health published a biography, Adverse Effects of Aspartame, listing no less than 167 reasons to avoid it. That's good enough reason alone, but if it's not good enough for you, then consider this!

"Aspartame was not approved until 1981, in dry foods. For over eight years the FDA refused to approve it because of the seizures and brain tumors this drug produced in lab animals. The FDA continued to refuse to approve it until President Reagan (a friend of Searle, the manufacturer) took office and fired the FDA Commissioner who wouldn't approve it. Dr. Arthur Hull Hayes was appointed as commissioner. Even then there was so much opposition to approval that a Board of

Inquiry was set up. The Board said: "Do not approve aspartame". Dr. Hayes OVERRULED his own Board of Inquiry. Shortly after Commissioner Arthur Hull Hayes, Jr., approved the use of aspartame in carbonated beverages, he left for a position with G.D. Searle's Public Relations firm."
[Source: thanks to Dorway.com for this little tidbit]

Long-Term Damage from Aspartame

Aspartame appears to cause slow, silent damage in those unfortunate enough to not have immediate reactions and a reason to avoid it. It may take a year, or many years, but it seems to cause some reversible and some irreversible changes in health over long-term use.

Methanol or wood alcohol is a deadly poison, yet it comprises 10% of aspartame. Methanol is gradually released in the small intestine when aspartame encounters the enzyme chymotrypsin. The absorption of methanol into the body is sped up considerably when free methanol is ingested. Anything heated above 86 degrees Fahrenheit or 30 Celsius breaks Methanol down into formic acid and formaldehyde in the body. Formic acid has been shown to inhibit oxygen metabolism. Formaldehyde is a deadly neurotoxin that accumulates in the body over long periods of time, but is released very slowly once absorbed. If you consume aspartame, in one sense you are preparing yourself in advance for your own funeral, because another name for formaldehyde is embalming fluid.

Many chronic diseases like psoriasis, which seem to appear suddenly, have actually been building in the body over many years. The troops of Desert Storm were fed large amounts of aspartame-sweetened beverages, which had been heated to over 86 degrees F. in the sun. Many returned home with numerous disorders similar to what has been seen in persons who have been poisoned by formaldehyde.

Reactions to aspartame have been officially reported to the EPA by the tens of thousands and involve more than 60 health complications including abdominal pain, blood sugar control problems, joint pain, migraines and weight gain, just to mention a few. Check the Resources section for more sources of information on this awful stealth food additive.

Conclusions about Aspartame

Aspartame is a toxic drug. The conclusion that can be drawn from the abundance of available information is that Aspartame doesn't belong in the body. It's not food and if it's needed in the production of certain food products, you don't need them either. Anyone who is using aspartame to control weight is always shocked to find that independent studies have shown that aspartame causes weight gain compared to people consuming the same product with real sugar. It's interesting to say the least. Find alternatives, they always exist. Keep in mind that is may take as long as two months for the accumulative effects of Aspartame to subside once you give it up.

Water! There's no avoiding it if you want to heal.

There might not be a more important topic in the entire program, especially for those who don't drink it. Many people don't drink *any* water, much less an amount that is satisfactory. Volumes have been written about water and for good reason. You've heard it before, but perhaps not in this context. What you need to know about water is quite simple, but you need to get the idea entrenched so that water becomes part of your daily life to the extent of 6 to 8 large glasses every single day. Nothing less will do. For those who don't like to drink water it must simply be said - get over it!

Maybe your water is not the best - it may have a bad taste, it may be chlorinated, hard, or otherwise be unappealing. With very few exceptions, you can overcome these obstacles. Buy water over-the-counter. Rent or buy a distiller. Put a filter on your water supply. In whatever way you have to do it, make sure you have enough water *in your body.* Here are some facts.

The body is composed of 75% water, and the brain is about 85%. That's a lot of water, so it must be important to us. When we evolved from sea-based life to land-based, a very sophisticated water-preservation system was needed for our bodies to continue to function and that system has resided in us to this day. All body functions are linked to the available supply of water. When we deprive ourselves of water, the body goes into a 'siege' state, and life at the cellular level literally dries up. The natural flow of bodily fluids is drastically curtailed, cells themselves discontinue to exchange fluid with the surrounding environment, and functions diminish. This includes nutrient transfer and organ function (elimination). The brain takes priority over all other body functions as the primary organ, and also because its water requirements are the greatest. The end result of this water deprivation is the diminishing of all bodily functions from waste disposal to nutrient supply to cell growth.

The availability of vast amounts of various other liquids in our society does not help matters. Coffee, alcohol, and soft drinks are not water, yet we substitute them for water whenever we are thirsty. The effect of caffeine or alcohol on the body is radically different than that of pure water. Why are there such a number of overweight people in our society? One reason is because they don't know when they are thirsty, and they also don't know the difference between fluids and water. In the absence of water, the body goes into a storage mode. We then feel thirsty, and reach for our favorite beverages. After years of doing this, our bodies are bloated and normal fluids are not circulating properly. An all-too-common solution today, especially among the elderly, is the use of diuretics which are pharmaceuticals designed to eliminate water from our systems. This can be the opposite of what is required. One of the main ways we can retain water in our bodies is with the use of sodium (salt). With the exceptional and growing number of people today with high blood pressure, there are many (too many according to some) that avoid salt completely. We need salt, and the complete avoidance of it, medical emergencies aside, is not considered prudent.

Balance would seem to be the best course to take. Pure water in adequate amounts would seem to be in order. That way your body will be able to utilize whatever amount it requires, and naturally discard the rest through normal elimination channels. So what to do? - The natural thing. Drink lots of good water, eat well and let your body do the rest. In the healing of psoriasis, we want to take charge of the playing field - provide the correct environment and let your body do the healing. You will hear this again and again in this book.

Whole Food Nutrition

There is a support system being used by people who realize that getting more whole food nutrition into their systems is essential, but very difficult to do, especially given our current lifestyles. All medical authorities these days are recommending that we all get 5-9 servings (minimum) daily of fresh, raw fruits & vegetables in our diets. Yet most of us are unable to have even a couple of servings on average. A large part of our vegetables, for example, are either cooked, which kills the active enzymes in the food, or de-natured, which essentially means void of the vitamins and minerals that come with fresh food. This is aside from the fact that soil conditions today are often so poor that the essential nutrients are missing even before the plant is grown.

A method was developed in the last few years, reducing the essence of fresh produce to a powder form, which is then encapsulated. The result is many different fresh, raw and whole fruits & vegetables, salt & sugar removed, fiber and enzymes included. The secret to the success of this product is in the fact that the wholeness of the food is not disturbed in the process, and very low temperatures are used so as not to lose the nutrients.

Once the body begins to receive all of these nutrients on a routine, daily basis, it begins to purge itself of toxic waste. In other words, it has a similar effect as if you consumed the actual raw fruits & vegetables.

An option to supplementation is to take the time and effort to obtain and consume 10 servings of organic raw fruits & vegetables every day. Regardless, you should try to eat as many fresh raw fruits & vegetables as you can. If it's not a supplement, make sure you're dealing with organic fruits & vegetables. And don't kid yourself; getting 5-9 daily servings of fresh fruits & vegetables is no small feat. That's 35-64 servings a week!

The Life of Your Spine

Most people don't pay any attention to their spines until something goes wrong. Yours may be perfect. We do suggest, however, that you have it checked out and have a spinal adjustment made if indicated. The spine is extremely complicated, yet it takes very little to cause a disturbance.

The skin as an organ must receive electrical (nerve) energy to function. Each organ of the body receives stimulation from specific nerves extending out from the spinal column. If discs are out of place even slightly, disruption can take place. Nerve supply to the upper intestinal tract emanating from the mid-dorsal area of the spine can be affected. The direct link between the nerves of this area and the functioning of your intestines has long been established. In a study published by the American Osteopathic Association, lesions of the thoracic vertebrae were "followed by lowered strength, diminished elasticity and increased extensibility of the muscular walls of the stomach and *Intestines*".

Progressive deterioration of the discs can be a factor in nerve energy function. The soft material between the discs is first compressed, then extended, and finally the bones have thinned seriously and are fusing together. Nerve damage is almost inevitable. If this happens in the dorsal area, watch for digestive disturbances. The good news is that spinal adjustments can make a substantial difference to the proper positioning and therefore the functioning of your spine and all that it relates to in your digestive tract. Ask a chiropractor about it.

High Colonics

High colonics are a process of evacuating the large bowel completely. You may have already had one or more yourself. They are recommended as a cleansing and detoxifying method. Depending on where you live, it may not be possible to go to a clinic where colonics are provided, but there is an alternative and that is an intestinal cleansing program. Many of the measures you learned about so far can be considered cleansing activities, such as your improved eating habits, or taking whole food supplements, for example. Lecithin is considered to be cleansing to the arteries, preventing fatty deposits in their linings, and in that way assisting in detoxifying. As a reminder, high colonics can remove impacted materials from the colon, along with slow moving material that can leak back into your bloodstream, re-toxifying you. High colonics can give you a big jump in detoxification. You may want to try them if you haven't already. If you have no access to them, you may want to try a bowel-cleansing program, available in most health food stores. Check to make sure it is a program that is well recognized and has a track record. Some of these programs can take several weeks to do, so be prepared to make a commitment.

Again, the objective of this book is to help you to:

- Detoxify
- Change your habits
- Discontinue the consumption of toxins

The corresponding results to be expected from the three major adjustments above are:

- Self-awareness, or knowing what you're doing at all times
- Transformation of your cells and your being
- Wholeness, or being healed

Reality Check #8

Mother Nature is ready to heal you, but she can't do it alone. A grudging reluctance on your part is not enough. An Olympic athlete does not earn a gold medal their first time on the track, they must stay the course until the job is done. Your job is to get on the track and stay on it until *your* job is done. At that point you can make other decisions.

Chapter 9

The Importance & Relevance of Your Immune System

"It is not the physician who heals, but nature. All mankind needs for good health and healing is provided in nature. The challenge to science is to find it."
- Paracelsus (1493 – 1541)

For you to understand how it is that you continue to have psoriasis, a visit to the immune system is essential. Once you understand the basics of immunity, the work you have to do to clear your psoriasis will make much more sense to you, making the journey easier. It is the autoimmune aspect of psoriasis that causes so much confusion, even in medical circles.

Witness the following definition by the National Institutes of Health:

"Psoriasis is an immune system disorder that affects the skin, and occasionally the eyes, nails, and joints. Psoriasis may affect very small areas of skin or cover the entire body with a build-up of red scales called plaques. The plaques are of different sizes, shapes, and severity and may be painful as well as unattractive. Bacterial infections and pressure or trauma to the skin can aggravate psoriasis. Most treatments focus on topical skin care to relieve the inflammation, itching, and scaling. For more severe cases, oral medications are used. Psoriasis is common and may affect more than 2 out of 100 Americans. Psoriasis often runs in families."

It is astounding that with the acceptance of the fact that psoriasis is autoimmune in nature, we keep plastering creams and lotions on top, and never get to the bottom of it. As Paracelsus said, the challenge is for science to find the bottom. There does not appear to be a concerted effort within most of the medical community to work with Mother Nature to do the very thing required in the circumstances, which is to re-balance the immune system. There is, however, a rush to find new drugs, which if successful will nevertheless only address the symptoms, as with all drugs. It will be left up to you to find the right approach, but the good news is that you have the tools right now.

Let's cover the basics of the immune system in order to clarify for you just how it is that psoriasis is allowed to continue in the body - unnecessarily.

On a day-to-day basis, your immune system is the only thing standing between you and certain death. Our physical and emotional health is governed by our immune systems, which is a complex network of white blood cells, immune co-factors, and antibodies protect our bodies from infection by foreign invaders of all kinds.

A State of Ready Alert

In days of antiquity, doctors knew that people who recovered from the plague would never get the disease again because they had acquired immunity against it. From there the concept of the immune system's 'memory' was borne. White blood cells have this astounding ability; you should be thankful for it since it keeps you alive daily. This is the same principle used in modern day vaccination programs, as controversial as they may be. The bottom line is that your immune system needs to be in a 'state of ready alert' when pathogens come calling. The best way to accomplish this is to foster a healthy lifestyle. The simplicity of this fact escapes many people, who constantly look in the wrong direction – externally – for the answers. The real answers are within you, in the nurturing of the cells of your body, particularly the cells of your intestines, where precious nutrient exchange takes place.

The key to a functional immune system is its ability to tell the difference between self and non-self. The ability to discriminate between normal activity in the body and foreign particles like bacteria, viruses, and toxins is the key. People with psoriasis have an additional problem due to leaky gut syndrome. The foreign particles in this case also come from food, macromolecules large enough to be recognized by the immune system as invaders. This sets up an autoimmune response.

Here's what happens. Antigens are specific surface molecules on all cells that identify them. If they are 'self' the immune system ignores them. If not, then antibodies are released by the immune system to fight them. Micronutrients from food are absorbed into the bloodstream, and pass inspection because they are broken down into particles small enough to be put to use in providing energy to healthy cells. Macronutrients on the other hand, do not belong in the blood due to their large size, so they become the enemy and are attacked as antigens. Not only viruses, bacteria, toxins, fungi, and parasites qualify as foreign, but also the very food you eat which more often than not comes with an array of toxins from herbicides, pesticides, and food additives.

The Key is Balance

The immune system is an extremely complex network of trillions of white blood cells called lymphocytes. The white blood cells in the body have abilities to perform specific tasks, but certain factors either limit that ability or impair its effectiveness. This in turn can affect the appropriateness of the immune response. With psoriasis, there is an inflammatory response causing a skin reaction. Research is ongoing to try to determine how regulatory T-cells fit into the psoriasis picture. T-cells are called regulatory because their job is to basically turn other immune cells in the immune complex on and off. When T-cells go rampant, you can have a type of runaway condition, and your skin cells proliferate too quickly. This is not to be confused with psoriasis, which has always been defined as proliferation of skin cells. It draws attention away from the real definition of psoriasis which is an autoimmune disorder caused by leaky gut. In one way of looking at it, your problem really isn't your skin; it's your leaky gut. Repair that, and you stop the autoimmune response because there will be no food-related antigens to attack.

A new drug therapy for psoriasis has been trotted out in 2003, but before you get all excited, take notice. It targets and suppresses T-cell activity in the hopes of preventing the inflammatory response. Not only is it extremely expensive (about $85 a day), it comes with strong warnings about the potential dangers of interfering with the immune system. And so it should. Drugs are a choice that people make in the treatment of psoriasis, yet they are becoming the choice of too many medical practitioners who are unprepared to take the more difficult, but effective, road to natural healing.

Underactive vs. Overactive (your type)

Underactive immune systems may be caused by heredity, chemotherapy, emotional stress, excessive exercise, poor nutrition, surgery, accidents, or aging. This can lead to infections or illnesses that we would otherwise toss off in the normal course of being healthy. AIDS patients are a case in point. It is all too often that the increased susceptibility from a breakdown in their immune systems allows for opportunistic infections to take root, causing their death.

An underactive immune system is not your problem, however. It is an *overactive* immune system that you are dealing with.

Overactive immune systems produce autoimmune conditions of all kinds, including psoriasis. Very common allergies are usually nothing more than an immune system overreacting to things like pollen or animal dander. Allergies are quite common among psoriatics. Other autoimmune conditions are arthritis, multiple sclerosis, lupus, certain types of diabetes, fibromyalgia, and colitis. Immune system suppressive drugs are frontline treatments for these conditions. Taking natural healing information seriously will help you avoid the tragedy of drug-based treatments.

Immunity and Leaky Gut

At least 70% of all antibody-producing cells are located in our digestive system, making more antibodies than any other cells in the body. You can imagine what happens when the delicate balance of organisms comprising the gut lining are disturbed or even destroyed. The very home of the immune system is made ineffectual. The hundreds of probiotics (friendly bacteria) residing in the gut are either destroyed or overcome by unwanted bacteria. While your immune system is busy attempting to repair itself, other areas of the body needing its attention are left to fend for themselves. The obvious result of this neglect is further degeneration of the body until the situation is rectified. Of course, with many people the situation is never rectified as they continue to pour in the toxins, creating a never-ending cycle of destruction to the gut lining and to their overworked immune systems. In these cases, you can almost expect a cascade of various health problems, like psoriatic arthritis for example.

Antibodies are to be found in your gut, or just moving around with your bloodstream. The antibodies produced in the gut do not cross the digestive tract walls nor can those in the blood get into our digestive tract. Remember that the digestive tract is 'outside' the body. For this reason, we need 'resident' antibodies to deal with the nastiness of what we consume every day, even from so-called good food.

Inflammatory Responses

When skin is damaged as with psoriasis, an immune response called inflammation happens. The typical redness and swelling of psoriasis is familiar to most, yet most don't think of psoriasis as inflammation. Cells of the immune system migrate into 'sites' of psoriasis as commanded by chemical messengers, or immune co-factors. Other white blood cells have released these co-factors as part of the overall immune response.

It is the overactivity of the immune system over a long period of time that results in inflammatory conditions producing the autoimmune aspect of psoriasis. Once you get your mind around this concept, things will begin to change for you, and you can begin to take corrective action. The medical hexing of psoriasis as an incurable disease of unknown origin leaves too many people stranded and feeling hopeless. This will hopefully come

to an end as more and more people find a better way –
healing the gut and balancing the immune system.

The Antibiotic Factor

Antibiotics are over prescribed drugs that are used to kill
unfriendly bacteria. Sadly, many doctors prescribe them
for viral conditions, upon which they have no effect. The
problem begins when friendly bacteria are taken out
with the offending bacteria, leaving an opportunity for
hundreds of species of unwanted bacteria to multiply
and mutate at will. Mutated bacteria grow stronger and
are known as antibiotic-resistant bacteria. This is
becoming a huge problem that you can avoid by asking
questions of your doctor before taking them. Ask if
antibiotics are really necessary in the instance, and what
repercussions there might be for you if you don't take
them, particularly in the light of your psoriasis.

Creating a Balanced Immune System

Helping yourself to a more balanced immune system is
not rocket science. You need to eat better, exercise, and
apply principles of natural healing to the greatest extent
possible. Eat lots of fresh fruits & vegetables, in raw
form whenever possible. When that's difficult, as it is for
90% of people, look to whole food supplementation (See
Reference section for source of supply).

Exercise should be moderate because heavy, prolonged
exercise like marathons produces too many free radicals
unless you have something powerful to counterbalance
them with. Commitment is the key word, consistently
doing the right things day after day until you have
control.

Reality Check #9

How's your immune system? Do you suffer from colds or
the flu several times a year? This is a clear sign of an
unbalanced immune system. There is no reason to have
a cold – ever! How about aching joints? This is not a
normal part of life. It may be time for you to examine
your life from the point of view of your susceptibility to
general illness. It would make for a good start.

Chapter 10

Last Rites for the Old Food Chain

"We have a situation where the very companies that stand to profit are the ones who decide whether or not their products are hazardous."
- John Robbins, author of 'The Food Revolution'.

Is food an important element in reversing psoriasis or not? The resounding answer is yes! – It's beyond dispute. Food is in fact the greatest detoxification agent known. If you accept the fact that psoriasis is a state of 'unwell', then anything contributing to a state of general health will be of help. So let's assume for the time being that if your general health were to improve, your psoriasis would improve as well, and we'll proceed from there.

Optimal Health is a term being used these days. Many people feel they are in good health, only to be shocked to learn from their doctor that the opposite is the case. Why? Because we are trained in our society for crisis intervention, not prevention. A great number of people are in a state of denial about their general health. Just ask your doctor. Optimal health is the elevation of not only general health, but of the awareness of It. Do you recall your days of youthful vigor? Can you even remember that push of energy? Health is so much more than the absence of disease, and we must strive to change our focus.

Many years ago there was an expression "You are what you eat". That expression has been modified in the light of modern research into food chemicals, and it now reads, "You are what you absorb". This means that life exists at the cellular level, and it is at this level that health begins and ends. It is the exchange of nutrients between the blood and the cells that creates the energy of life. Researchers have found that the elements of food known as phytochemicals, of which there are more than 10,000 and counting, are instrumental at the cellular level of our bodily functions. No one seriously suggests that food and health are not related; yet many would argue that your diet is not a factor at all in psoriasis. There are even those who state that psoriasis has no connection to toxicity, rather it is the result of genetics. Although genetics may play a role in *propensity*, it is not the governing factor. In the meantime, we may choose to work with what we know can make a significant difference in our health - our food intake.

Take to heart the words of some of the experts below:

Dr. Hari Sharma, M.D. – author of 'Free Radicals'
"A growing consensus in society indicates that the basic premises of modern health care may need revising. The allopathic approach waits for symptoms of disease to arise, then brings to bear a vast armory of machinery, drugs, surgical procedures, and hospital equipment to fight the symptoms and/or the causes as they appear. The most tragic aspect of the modern approach, however, is that the allopathic system is itself a major cause of ill health and disease. The side effects of drugs are notoriously damaging, especially if many drugs are prescribed simultaneously. There could be a simple solution to all of this, if only it were possible: ideally we would be able to prevent illness before it begins. Unfortunately, keeping people healthy has appeared a daunting task. Exercise and diet control have been proven effective, but it is hard to get people to change their habits."

Michael T. Murray, N.D. – author of 'Dietary and Lifestyle Recommendations for Psoriasis'.
"Consume a diet that focuses on whole, unprocessed foods (whole grains, legumes, vegetables, fruits, nuts, and seeds). Avoid animal products with the exception of cold-water fish (salmon, mackerel, herring, halibut, etc.). Identify and control food allergies, and eliminate alcohol, caffeine, and sugar. Get regular exercise, and perform a relaxation exercise 10 to 15 minutes each day. Drink at least 48 ounces of water daily."

James F. Balch, M.D. & Phyllis A. Balch, C.N.C.
- authors of 'Prescription for Nutritional Healing'.
"When we do not give ourselves the proper nutrients, we can cause great harm to the body by impairing its

normal functions. The problem with most of us is that we do not get what we need from our "modern diet". Even if you are not sick, you may not necessarily be healthy. It simply may be that you are not yet exhibiting any overt symptoms of illness. [Editorial note: Not the case with psoriasis] By understanding the principles of holistic nutrition, and knowing what nutrients we need, we can improve the state of our health, stave off disease, and maintain a harmonious balance in the way nature intended."

To enter into a full discussion of the problems inherent in our modern day system of food delivery would take a few dozen books. Our main thrust in this chapter is simply to turn on a few lights in this very dark room called 'food processing'. It is important for you to have an understanding of how modern food production works so that you can make more informed decisions about your own food choices. Moreover, you will begin to see that there are economic forces at play that could care less about the state of your health. Of more significance to them is the state of their balance sheets. When jobs are on the line, altruistic motivations move to the background. Our food is being de-natured faster than we can track it. McDonalds, for example, who make some of the unhealthiest fast foods, are tweaking their menus to gain the slightest competitive advantage over other fast food outlets by introducing 'healthier' French fries. This came about mainly as a result of considerable public pressure, not because of healthier attitudes amongst the corporate executives. As you begin to see the reality of how corporate America treats our food supply, begin to read labels, and listen closely to the advertisements, you will gain power over your subconscious, which is where the marketing efforts go. No longer will you automatically reach for that food item; first you'll look, then analyse, and only then will you either buy or walk away.

The extremely effective marketing techniques used by the food giants have now passed through a few generations and are well entrenched in our subconscious. Our children, in spite of meagre attempts to educate them in ways of healthy eating, are overcome by the media onslaught of crass

108

merchandising without regard to any health issues. Have
you ever watched a TV ad, only to ask at the end of it –
'What was that for?' This is because the ad was directed
at your subconscious, not your conscious mind. The real
message was not about the product, but about how
'good' you're going to feel the next time you buy it on
impulse without really knowing why.

Generation Degeneration

The consequences of marketing bad food products are
truly daunting. It is predicted that as the baby boomers
go into their sixties and hit the medical system hard,
they will bring it to its knees. What's worse, the
generation of former 'kids' who are now reaching thirty
will cross with the boomers in the corridors of hospitals
with the same problems, creating utter chaos. Imagine
sixty-somethings and thirty-somethings having the
same problems. This could only be called 'generation
degeneration'. Each generation is getting worse, and
faster than the last. Research reveals that fully 40% of
children at age 12 display some signs of coronary heart
disease. The projections are scary.

Your body is comprised of roughly 60 trillion cells, each
one of which can mutate or die without the nutrition
they need. When you think about it, your genetics have
passed down uninterrupted throughout history since the
dawn of man millions of years ago. This is the miracle
DNA plan that was created for us. If your lineage had
faltered just once in the last two million years, you
would not be here. It is shocking to realize that it is only
in the last 50 or 60 years that we have begun to mess
with our genetic makeup through the use of modern
food processing, introducing thousands upon thousands
of chemical additives to our food chain, and de-naturing
food in order to create longer shelf life thereby
increasing profits for multinational corporations.

Our DNA can be maintained quite simply, but in today's
world it has become quite a task to sort things out, but
you can do it. All you need is quality food, water, air,
and light. The first three have been so badly
contaminated that many of us now take it for granted
yet we still have power over how we manage them. To

return to a state of natural health takes three constant steps:

1) Do not apply poisons to your DNA structure. This includes toxic drugs, chemicals, radiation from many sources, smoking, alcohol, and processed foods.
2) Present the *proper* building blocks to your multi-million-year-old genetic program, namely food, water, air and light.
3) Ensure that your digestive system works well, or you will toxify and defeat everything else. Remember, it's not just what you eat that matters, but what you *absorb*. Proper absorption of nutrients only takes place in a healthy digestive tract.

At the turn of the century, most people still ate from gardens. Their ancestors passed down simple gardening techniques that were used without herbicides and pesticides. This has all but disappeared, beginning with the advent of canned food decades ago. Nowadays, we accept most of what we hear, and we hear lots, especially compared to the turn of the century when not even radio was available to the masses.

Let's bring up a few examples and see which ones surprise you.

- Calcium, silicon, zinc, and selenium are lost when distilled water is consumed. These are major cancer fighters.

You are targeted: *We have been convinced* to buy distilled water because our regular supply is not adequate.

Tip: Filter your water at home with a filter that leaves the mineral content intact, but removes the chlorine. When buying water, buy only re-mineralized water.

- Hydrogenated margarine was 'invented' around 1910. Chemists found a way to bubble hydrogen gas into liquid vegetable oil which was then heated to a high temperature. Nickel when added helps as a catalyst, and food colouring is added to 'enhance' the colour of the margarine. If you are old enough to remember, margarine used to come with small packets of colouring powder that you mixed into the whitish blob of hydrogenated fat that we call a butter substitute.

You are targeted: *We have been convinced* that margarine is a safer bet than butter because of the fat content of butter. The real reason for this promotion is that hydrogenated products are cheap, stable, and have a long shelf life. It's economics once again. Rather than the product having a long shelf life, we want *you* to have a long shelf life.

Tip: Watch for the word 'hydrogenated' on packaging, and avoid hydrogenated products altogether.

- Most of the cholesterol circulating in our blood is made in our own bodies by the liver. The lesser portion is consumed, and the 'culprits' are indicated as eggs, meats, and butterfat among other things. These do not in themselves increase blood cholesterol. Dr. Atkins, notable for his controversial diet consisting partially of protein consumption, is currently being redeemed in some studies. Of more significance to your cholesterol may be simple sugar, a refined carbohydrate that elevates blood fats and triglycerides. These are three fatty acids that come from a glycerol molecule that is produced by the liver under conditions of excess sugar. High glycemic-index foods like raw sugar increase blood sugar content at too fast a rate for your system to handle.

You are targeted: *We have been convinced* to eliminate cholesterol from our diets or to avoid it completely. That's why you see 'Cholesterol-free' on products that never contained cholesterol in the first place. Marketing!

Tip: Avoid any product that has these words on the label - sugar, corn syrup, corn starch, maltodextrin, dextrose, glucose, white flour, and white rice. They all contribute to glucose overload and the problems discussed above. As you read labels, make note of the fact that ingredients are listed in their order of dominance. Sugar is all too often the number one or number two listed ingredient.

- According to Dr. Humbart Santillo, N.D. (author of Intuitive Eating), meat contains 14 times more pesticides than plant foods, and dairy contains 5.5 more times. Chemicals in our food may cause allergies, digestive problems, asthma, and skin problems like psoriasis and eczema, and fatigue symptoms. The elimination of eggs, meat and dairy will often alleviate the problem.

You are targeted: *We have been convinced* by the Food Guides to eat damaging foods we can do without if we are prepared to educate ourselves properly.

Tip: Moderation is still the key. You have to decide how much or how little meat you are willing to have in your diet. One thing's for sure – you don't need dairy products to get your calcium, and you don't need the toxins concentrated in meats like chicken and beef to get your proteins.

- A main staple of our North American diet is bread, particularly white bread. White bread was originally considered almost a delicacy enjoyed by the upper classes. It was indeed delicate, almost melting in the mouth, and no wonder! Naturally the main ingredient in white bread is white flour, but most people don't know how white flour comes about. Here's the short story, and a sad one it is. White flour begins as whole wheat flour. The bran and germ is removed and passed along, unbelievably, mostly for animal food. The best part of the food goes to animals. The flour is then bleached with chlorine gas, eliminating vital nutrients that remain. The end product is void of nutrients. This is the reason that health officials have forced companies to 'enrich' breads with certain nutrients like niacin and thiamine, along with partially hydrogenated vegetable shortening. The name of the game is extending the shelf life. The mass marketers of bread products brag about the life span of their products.

You are targeted: *We have been convinced* that bread, especially white bread, should be a part of our daily diets, whereas the very opposite is true. Bulky foods without fibre or nutrition slow the digestive tract and cause problems.

Tip: Minimize bread consumption and recognise its various forms. Find alternatives for the meals where you are tempted to make a bread-type meal. Know that bread is a very high glycemic-index food that causes your pancreas to secrete insulin to combat the high sugar levels caused by bread consumption.

French Fries - Fun Food?

Consider this; there are some unregulated restaurants that keep their French fry oils for weeks before changing them. Even with regular inspections, it is difficult for inspectors to know how long oil is kept. Often the rule of thumb is for the staff to demand an oil change in the kitchen because of the terrible odor. Oil at high temperature gets rancid very quickly, especially when several menu items are cooked in the same oil every day. At night the oil is cooled and first thing in the morning it is turned on again to reach the boiling point for the next 12-20 hours. The cycle continues until someone makes the decision to change it. That decision is an economic one because oil costs money. The next time you are tempted to have French fries in a restaurant, ask the server what kind of oil is used. Most won't know, but you have a right to know, it's going into your body, and you're paying for it. Be prepared for the answer to shock you, but know your oils. The best strategy is to never have another French fry in your life.

Educate Yourself - It's Free!

Sounds simple enough. The problem is to make the
commitment. Some people don't even like to read.
That's a problem, but it's one that can be overcome. No
one is asking you to become a *reader.* But if you're
serious about ridding yourself of psoriasis, some degree
of exploration is required. No matter what the discussion
is about, people will not commit to do anything until *it
makes sense* to them. Pick up magazines and look for
articles that you think apply to health or psoriasis in
some way. Make slight changes on what you find that
makes sense to you. Look for books in libraries or
bookstores on subjects that may help you. Check the
Internet, it's loaded. Ask people you know who are
'health nuts' (you don't have to become one).

Read food labels

This can be a very powerful ally indeed if used properly,
and the way to use it properly is to do it all the time,
even with food products that you think you know well.
You'll be surprised. There is a cat-and-mouse game that
is played out in the food industry with labels vs. the
government (FDA in the U.S. or the Department of
Consumer Affairs in Canada, for example).
Manufacturers usually try to 'dress up' their ingredient
list so that it reads well to the consumer, and in many
cases alternative names are used to disguise the basic
ingredient. Sugar is a classic, with many names being
used in place of 'sugar'. Get to know them.

Ingredients are listed in order of quantity on food labels.
You'll notice sugar appearing in first or second spot a
lot, for example. That should scare you away. The
companies making the products would not put the
ingredients on the label if it weren't the law. Food labels
are very revealing, and if you're not used to them,
they're confusing as well, but you do get on to it. You
may need a dictionary at first or a food guide
pocketbook (sometimes found on supermarket
shelves!).

Why is elimination of some of the basic foods you eat
every day recommended? Unless you're very young,

your enzyme capacity has diminished, and whereas white breads, starches and cooked foods never used to be a problem for you, they are now. The main reason is that these same foods can cause constipation, blood diseases, bleeding ulcers, bloating, and arthritis. As you age, the enzyme content of the body depletes, and food is not properly digested. It ferments and produces the toxins that are then absorbed into the blood and deposited in the joints and other soft-tissue areas, bringing on illness you never knew before.

What's in a Label?

You really have to educate yourself as to labels and their true meaning. Here are a few tips, and they are just the "tip" of the iceberg when it comes to food labeling. Get a good book on the subject. Make no mistake, the companies that use bad ingredients in their products for reasons of taste or shelf life are playing games with the regulators, plus they are trying to trick you. It works unless you're educated to labeling.

Food Industry Words Used: Reduced Fat
Regulatory Intent: 25 to 33% less fat than normal
Reality: Still very fatty
Examples: Cheese, margarine, sour cream, dairy

Food Industry Words Used: Cooked in Vegetable Oil
Regulatory Intent: Poly or mono-unsaturated (good!)
Reality: May be palm oil (50% saturated – very bad)
Examples: Any that say 'hydrogenated'

Food Industry Words Used: 97% Fat Free
Regulatory Intent: None, it's just a marketing ploy
Reality: 97% Fat Free
Examples: Does not mean 97% **less** fat

Food Industry Words Used: Lite (light)
Regulatory Intent: Low in calories
Reality: Lightly "salted" but same amount of fat
Examples: Potato chips, beer, light olive oil, light cake

Exercise caution & avoid buying foods with these terms on the packaging:

Artificial Colorings, aspartame, BHA & BHT (package preservatives), Quinine, Artificial flavoring, MSG (monosodium glutamate), Sulphites (sodium bisulphite, sulphur dioxide), Acesulfame Potassium, Cyclamate, Olestra (Olean), Saccharin, Sodium Nitrate, Sodium Nitrite (all processed meats).

Avoiding these terms will automatically eliminate a lot of food from your diet, but there's still a whole bunch left.

Enzymes – Without Which Nothing Takes Place

Here is how Dr. Humbart Santillo, author of 'Intuitive Eating', defines an enzyme:

"Let me clarify this by giving you an example: a light bulb can only light up when you put an electric current through it. It is animated by electricity. The current is the life force of the bulb. Without electricity we would have no light, just a light bulb. So we can say that the light bulb actually has a dual nature; a physical structure and a non-physical electrical force that expresses and manifests through the bulb. The same situation exists when trying to describe what an enzyme is within our body structure. Each enzyme acts in certain ways in the body doing specific jobs such as digesting food, building protein in the bones and skin, and aiding detoxification. Once we cook at high temperatures though, the enzyme is destroyed. It no longer carries on its dedicated function. Although the physical protein is still present, it has lost its life force."

Thus we can see that the electrical energy that used to drive our resources is no longer present in adequate levels to get the job of **digestion and building skin**. In short, enzymes are what count, and we would be well advised to do whatever it takes to keep them in place.

What Happens with Too Few Enzymes

If you lack the necessary enzymes, food particles can pass undigested into the bloodstream. The body's immune system identifies the particles as foreign, and attacks with antibodies. The resulting effect is allergy, inflammation, and in your case psoriasis. Remember, you already have thinner intestinal walls to start with. You need more enzymes, and the older you are, the more you need because the body's ability to provide its own enzymes decreases with age. Enzymes are found in fresh foods, especially raw fruits & vegetables. All 'live' food comes with it's own enzymes for digestion.

Maybe you've been doing it all along. Let's hope so. Here are some topics to cover, which may present a challenge to you beyond what you've had so far. Just remember the goal - *control* over your psoriasis. *Relief* can be purchased at the drug store. Here we're on to something more meaningful.

The 7-day Food List Challenge!
Self-monitor your food intake for a week.

Carry a small notebook with you everywhere you go for a week. Take the time each day to mark down everything that goes in your mouth for the next 7 days. Everything! - water, food of any kind, drinks, snacks - *everything.* Within the first couple of days you will surprise yourself not only with what you consume, but what you consume unconsciously. This simple exercise can really be beneficial in waking you up to your habits. Keep going for a whole week, even though you think it's kind of silly. At the end of the week, sit yourself down and read over your list. It's a real eye-opener.

Food Additives

Labeling and food additives comprise a very large subject. Food additives in our modern marketplace are almost a necessary evil in order to keep goods on grocery store shelves and to transport them long distances, but it doesn't mean you have to eat them. It is a matter of philosophy as to how the world should change to either get back to "the old days" or to grow food regionally in order to keep it fresh. Having said that, there is much you can do the get away from these nasty things. You don't have to be a part of it, at least not to any great degree. Additives make our soft drinks sweet without sugar, and they keep our bread from going moldy. One prominent bread company prides itself on their bread still being soft after **one month!** The view from here is, 'if it looks like bread, and smells like bread, that doesn't mean it's bread'. Other clever phrases used in food processing trick you into believing that you're buying real food. *Fruit-flavored* has nothing to do with fruit. *Chicken taste* doesn't mean chicken. *Cranberry drink* doesn't mean cranberry juice. Even if it did contain real juice, a 5% mix of real cranberry juice can validate the manufacturer's claim that the jar contains real cranberry juice.

Self-education is the answer to this marketplace. Many food additives have been declared safe after much testing, others have not but are still permitted. It is often a roll of the dice. Our advice is for you to become one of the people who are informed about these matters. It gives you great power over what you take into your body, and the less additives you consume the more energy your body has to get Job #1 done, the healing of your psoriasis. Fewer toxins, more progress. Everything that goes into your mouth is a choice - make it a conscious one every time.

Reality Check #10

What is the extent of your food knowledge? Do you scrutinize labeling on food products, or do you just throw them in your shopping basket? It may be time that you got involved in what's going into your mouth, and the only way is to begin a slow, steady education. You may not like what you learn, but you will be an empowered consumer in the end.

Chapter 11

The Case for Supplementation

"It is not to the credit of my profession that we are so late in discovering that nutrition is one key to healing. However, even that changes, albeit so slowly. When the medical profession finally discovers nutrition you will see advances in preventive health care the likes of which have never before occurred." – Gary Price Todd, M.D.

In a way it is unfortunate that this chapter even has to be written, but general awareness is not yet high enough to leave it out. Not only that, unbelievably there still remain many people who have yet to be exposed to the flood of information on supplementation and its ramifications for general health. In our modern society, supplementation is no longer an option for anyone who has even a minimal understanding of current health matters. We have an epidemic of obesity in North America for starters. With 40% of our youth now considered to be obese, something has to be done. We are the most overfed and undernourished people on earth, which is quite a thing when you consider the resources we have on hand. The trouble is that it's our resources that are creating the problem. While the vast majority of the world is still cultivating the ground, we have developed highly sophisticated manufacturing facilities that quite literally mass-produce and box our food for us. It's a totally hands-free set-up as far as the consumer is concerned. All we have to do is show up with the money.

We already know we are overfed. That's what Weight Watchers was built on – calorie counting. What many people are unaware of is that at the same time that we are overfed, we are undernourished. That means that although we are getting bulk, it is so depleted of nutrients that our bodies are actually starving. It's no wonder that we put on weight. Our bodies think we are going to die, and go into starvation mode, literally 'putting food away' for a rainy day. That rainy day never comes, though, since day after day for years we continue to have our three square meals, plus snacks!

Food has become entertainment, and entertainment is food. We can't see a movie or attend a sporting event without it. Advertisers inundate us with new products, touting sugar products in the early morning, getting our systems all revved up and ready for the mid-morning donut. It's madness.

In the midst of all of this, we are expected to cope. It's not working. In order to survive our modern world, with its glut of choices, we have to take ourselves out of the picture. It would be a good idea for everyone to sit down and make up their own list of acceptable foods, as extensive and variable as they wish to make it. When complete, they could refer to it when faced with food choices. This would really simplify things in the advertising world – if it's not on your list, it doesn't get any attention. And don't think you'd be missing out, either. Any company that has the millions to advertise will make sure that they get their product in your face sooner or later, and if they don't, you can bet a friend of yours will. Consumers are the pinballs of marketing, but need to take back control. These companies are not your friends.

What supplementation is, and what it is not

Supplementation is not the answer to bad food habits. If Twinkies are your mainstay, all is lost. No amount of vitamins or minerals will compensate for the damage done by consuming bad food year upon year. So supplements are meant to do what their name implies – supplement! It is essential to make changes in your diet according to the program you are following, and then find the right supplements to add to quality foods.

Supplementation is the addition of nutrients to your body beyond food intake. They 'top up' your nutritional requirements rather than neutralize your bad choices. There is a huge difference in perspective here, and you need to truly understand this simple principle. Multivitamins are not the antidote for beer, and vitamin

C is not the antidote for a cold. It is what can keep you from getting a cold in the first place.

The RDA (Recommended Daily Allowance) of nutrients that you find on food packaging is by some reports a joke. It has even been called the 'recommended death allowance', so pitifully deficient it is as a means of more than mere survival. It is no wonder that so many middle aged people limp through the day complaining of aches and pains, not to mention severe fatigue. Their bodies are suffering degenerative processes due to lack of proper nutrition. Our medical system has us completely convinced that should anything go wrong, they will be there to 'fix us'. The majority of people still believe that, although it is slowly changing, as more people find out that as Tiger Woods' father once said to him, "it's easy to check into the hospital, but real hard to check out."

If you are one of those who have vague illness, or simply lack that feel-good thing, or maybe you have chronic fatigue on top of your psoriasis, it's time you sat yourself down and had a talk about supplementation. Degraded food products, nutrient-free foods, depleted soils, sugar-dominated food substitutes, rancid-oil-laden treats and desserts, and a myriad of other substances that add up to a virtual assault on the modern human body, means that it's wake up time. This wasn't happening at the turn of the last century, a mere one hundred years ago on a planet that has been home to mankind for a couple of million years. Our modern processed foods were born a half-second ago on the million-year clock.

Supplements you need, and supplements to consider

1.   You *do need* a whole food supplement.

The prime reason is that you are likely among the 90% of North Americans that don't get 5-9 servings of fresh, raw fruits and vegetables every day. Another reason is that the 'fresh' food you may be buying is up to 90% void of nutrients, for reasons we have already mentioned. If you don't believe you need to supplement, do this simple test:

For one week, do the Food List Challenge. Write down everything that goes into your mouth. At the end of the week, add up the servings of fresh, raw fruits & vegetables you ate. A serving is roughly a half-cup.

You should be getting, minimally, 35 combined servings per week. Optimally, 63 servings. It's a test worth taking.

Note: it is not recommended to 'juice' whole foods in a juice machine, unless you
    1) Have a lot of time on your hands
    2) Can buy pure organic foods
If organic foods are not available to you, and you still choose to juice, just remember that you're concentrating herbicides and pesticides into a six-ounce glass. It's not a wise choice, and has far too much sugar, especially for someone with psoriasis.

If supplementation in this area makes sense to you, check the Resources Section in this book for a source of whole food supplements in capsules, sugar and salt removed.

2.   You may wish to *consider* a calcium supplement.

One reason is that calcium is an essential for bodily functions. Not only that, but calcium is highly alkaline, a real benefit for psoriasis. Basically, healthy people are slightly alkaline, and ill people are acidic. Cancer is highly acidic, for example.

When it comes to selecting a calcium supplement, quality is paramount. For one thing, Vitamin D is not only important, but also essential for calcium absorption; do not buy any calcium product that has not addressed that issue.

Whether or not you continue to take calcium beyond your psoriasis healing is a personal choice. Many take it to counter the effects of osteoporosis, yet resistance training (small weight lifting) is considered by many to be just as valuable to prevent calcium loss. This is a different issue than supplementing, because calcium is

constantly required in the process of the proper
exchange of energy at the cellular level of the body.

3.   If you take a vitamin supplement....

If you don't take a whole food supplement, which is by
far preferable, then you'll be missing the vitamins that
come in whole foods, and you may need to consult with
a professional to make proper decisions. Vitamins are
not harmless, and some consider them drugs. Because
they can throw off the body's balance when taken as an
isolated substance, they should only be taken if a
deficiency is known, and only after consideration. Some
people are already taking multivitamins, and won't
consider anything else, but they should. The biggest
percentage of vitamins ingested are not taken up into
the bloodstream, but flushed down the toilet. That's 90
cents out of every dollar. Your financial advisor would
likely frown on that. Vitamins are second best to raw
fruits & vegetables, the original source of many
vitamins. Vitamins are black & white TV compared to the
colour TV of fresh fruits & vegetables.

4.   You *do need* Essential Fatty Acid (EFA)
      supplementation. They have a modulating effect
      on the immune system, govern genes for fat
      metabolism, and cannot be manufactured by the
      body. That's why they're called 'essential'. Look
      to Chapter 8 for a detailed explanation and check
      the Resources section for ordering sources.

Reality Check #11

How seriously have you considered supplementation?
Vitamins are one thing, but the supplementation
discussed here is something else altogether. You've no
doubt taken some prescription medications before. It's
time to consider natural products. Some very serious
medical researchers and practitioners are absolutely
convinced that they are the future of medicine. That's
why many supplements are called 'nutriceuticals'
nowadays.

Chapter Twelve

Getting Down to Doing the Healing

"There are no short cuts. The map to psoriasis healing is a well-defined road, not a field to run around in".
- Author

Most people simply want to know what exactly to do, and why wouldn't they? But don't make the mistake of skipping to this chapter and just 'doing it'. A house without a foundation will not stand long, and this book is all about giving you a foundation of understanding that can last a lifetime. You need *reasons* for doing this work. Because of the horrendous way that psoriasis has been treated and explained in our society, you could almost call it a debriefing. If this is the first chapter you are seeing, go back and read the introduction and the previous chapters. There is plenty of time to get specific, but if you really want to start today, then start in this simple way – drink 6-8 glasses of pure water today, free of chlorine.

There are many components to a natural healing regimen. Each has been proven to add to the overall results, having come from nature itself. None are experimental, and none are dangerous, as with drugs. Each must be taken on its own merits, and added whenever possible to the daily routine. Some parts of the regimen will be more important to you than others; it depends very much on individual makeup.

The elements that make up a healing are:
1. Detoxification
2. Proper nutrition
3. Healing the intestinal tract
4. Balancing the immune system

These can be done simultaneously. For example, if you address all the components but still allow toxins to enter your system, you will likely not make any lasting progress.

Detoxification

This means purifying your blood by ridding it of accumulated toxins. To accomplish this, you need to provide relief to your organs, namely the liver, kidneys, lungs and ultimately, your skin, where your original psoriasis problem does not exist, but manifests. Detoxification through diet, exercise, and right living will purge your system of everything from pesticides to heavy metals. Some people go to great lengths to do this, up to and including chelation therapy, a sometimes expensive and time-consuming process. Proponents of chelation have very strong opinions regarding the effectiveness of the therapy, so if you choose to explore this possibility, it is recommended that you take you're time to research it well and get references. This is strictly a personal choice, but you should know that you could get the job done through diet and exercise on your own.

Proper Nutrition

This topic is covered elsewhere in the book, but suffice it to say that the best fresh, raw fruits & vegetables are absolutely fundamental to your healing. Aside from that, it is critical that you take to heart the recommendations for the additions as well as the deletions to your diet for as long as it takes you to heal.

Healing the Intestinal Tract

This will come about naturally as you change your diet, start to exercise, and begin to detoxify. As toxins disappear, your intestinal lining will return to the state that Mother Nature programmed it for, in the absence of all of the destructive forces that has overwhelmed it for so long.

Balancing the Immune System

Your immune system has been in overdrive for at least as long as you have had psoriasis. It is out of balance, and you are experiencing 'autoimmunity' when your immune system attacks the toxic invaders that have leaked into your bloodstream. Nothing will stop this process until you have taken the necessary steps to remove the invaders, so going back to the source of the problem – your diet – is paramount. Your immune system's natural state is balance, but it needs your full cooperation. The immune system is incredibly complex, but what you have to do to help it along is not.

The following are the do's and don'ts of food. Take these seriously and you're likely to see serious results. On the other hand, if you allow yourself 'exemptions' because of your obsessions with certain foods, you can expect poor results. Also remember that once you have achieved true healing, you can always add certain foods back into your diet on an experimental basis, but never sugar and white bread.

Mandatory Avoid List

1.   Raw sugar
2.   White bread/white flour
3.   Fatty & fried foods
4.   The Nightshade plants: tobacco, peppers (black table pepper is OK), eggplant, tomatoes, paprika, white potatoes
5.   All dairy products (get your calcium from vegetables or proper supplements)
6.   Too many acidic foods (20-30% maximum permitted to maintain acid/alkaline balance. See Chapter 6 for ratings)
7.   Soda pop & aspartame
8.   Alcohol of all kinds
9.   Caffeine – from coffee, tea, soda

Mandatory Do List

1.   Drink a minimum of 6-8 glasses of chlorine-free water daily. This facilitates the exchange of nutrients at the cellular level, and is essential for the removal of toxins. Without water, our cells 'lock up' and these processes come to a halt.

2.   Get aerobic exercise of your choice at least 3-4 times a week, daily if possible. The TV remote control doesn't count, and neither does your job, no matter what that might be. Walking does

count, as does swimming, exercise equipment, etc. It has been shown that the effects on metabolism last for several hours after exercise, plus the body detoxifies, and the lymphatic system is enervated.

3.   Eat 5-9 servings of fresh, raw fruits & vegetables daily – preferably organic. See Resources for high quality supplement options, free of sugar & salt. Fruits and vegetables are the very foundation of psoriasis healing. Do not cook them. Cooking destroys valuable nutrients and kills enzymes, placing more stress on your body.

4.   Have a cup of fresh squeezed lemon juice in hot water first thing in the morning or last thing before bed. This is a great cleanser as well as being highly alkaline.

5.   Take an enzyme supplement before each meal to help with breaking down nutrients. Otherwise, your body has to produce enzymes to get the job done, using up valuable resources in the process. Eating cooked foods for years on end will use up your lifetime supply of enzymes, which already deplete as you age. A good way to soften food is to lightly stream it using a steamer, but don't overdo it or you will get the same result as if you cooked it on the stove.

6.   Take two tablespoons of Omega 3/6 combination daily. You need both Omega 3 & Omega 6 essential fatty acids. They're called 'essential' because you need to obtain them from outside sources. Your health food store will be able to help.

7.   Take two tablespoons of granular lecithin daily. This can be mixed with juice or water. Make sure it's non-genetically modified. Lecithin is a good cleanser and fat emulsifier. A theory exists that psoriatics have difficulty with fat metabolism, but lecithin has value regardless.

8.   Find a meditation for peace of mind, the simpler the better. TV doesn't count, stargazing does. And of course there's real meditation, the best of all. Meditation lowers the heart rate, lowers blood pressure, and clears the mind of clutter. In other words, it gives you more peace, and who couldn't use more of that?

9.   You need to have a minimum of one bowel movement daily. Anything less means there is trouble somewhere. Two should be normal. If you are constipated, you need a diet change and more water, not drug store laxatives. Over a billion dollars a year are spent on laxatives, which can be damaging because some contain the chemical phenolphthalein, known to cause cancer. Besides, common 'remedies' can actually be habit-forming to the point where you must continue their use in order to have bowel movements. Increase your consumption of complex carbohydrates, meaning fruits & vegetables. Meat stays in the digestive tract up to 5 times as long as complex carbohydrates, and when it does, it putrefies.

10.   Try to do a random act of kindness every day. This means doing something 'nice' for someone with no strings attached. It's not a favour, because we usually expect favours to be returned. It can be something you do for a total stranger, as simple as letting someone into your traffic lane who looks stuck at an intersection. Or it can be something more significant like bringing a toy to a sick child. You'll think of things once you start doing it. The result will be that you not only 'feel better' but your immune system is stronger.

The **Daily Progress Chart** that follows can be used as your guide to success. Keep your book handy and mark the week's chart at the end of each day. You will be utterly surprised at what you learn about yourself and your habits after only a month of using it. After a couple of months you will start to see a pattern, which can help you to change some habits that you may not even have realized you had. It is both a visual and record-keeping way of seeing how you are progressing with the program. Keep each week's chart so that you can revisit periodically.

Because it is important for you to understand why it is that you are doing each item, a breakdown follows. Much of the explanation appears in other sections of the book, but for brevity's sake, here it is in one section.

Daily Progress Chart

Place an "x" in the box if completed for that day or leave blank. Give yourself 1 point for each box completed and total the day at the bottom. You will have a visual guide to your progress plus a point system. Do this for 6 months and you will clearly see your progress as well as your challenges.

After the first month, look at your 'Grand Totals' in the bottom right hand corner. Challenge yourself to gradually bring up the number.

PCI Daily Progress Chart
Summary Explanations
(See index for cross-references)

✓ **Water**
The essence of life, facilitating energy exchanges.
✓ **Aerobics**
Any kind to increase heart rate for 20-30 minutes.
✓ **Fruit**
Minimum of 3 servings of fresh fruit daily. (if you have Candida, skip this, or better - use supplements – see Resources)
✓ **Vegetables**
Minimum of 5 raw servings daily. Serving is a half-cup. (Supplement alternative – see Resources)
✓ **Alcohol**
None for now, perhaps moderately later after healing.
✓ **Raw sugar**
None of any kind - white, brown or otherwise.
✓ **Nightshades**
No tobacco, paprika, white potato, peppers, eggplant, tomato – bad chemistry for psoriasis.
✓ **Fried foods**
Destructive to digestive system, especially heated oils.

✓ **Soda**
None - phosphates in pop leach calcium from bones + sugar content is excessive.

✓ **Caffeine**
Negative effect on digestion – found mainly in coffee & soft drinks.

✓ **Acid/alkaline balance**
Refer to chart, keep ratio maintained (see page 82).

✓ **Dairy**
None – it is mucus forming & anti-cleansing.

✓ **White flour**
It is acid forming and de-natured. Eliminate it.

✓ **Smoking**
A 3000+ chemical assault on your system.

✓ **Lemon juice**
Highly alkaline & cleansing.

✓ **Enzymes**
Aid in digestion, takes burden off body's enzyme production.

✓ **Combination Omega 3 & 6 essential oils**
EFA's (essential fatty acids).

✓ **Lecithin**
Good for cleansing & fat emulsion (aids in fat metabolism)

✓ **Meditation**
Relaxes nervous system, de-stresses. See Resources.

✓ **Skin Brushing**
Stimulates lymph, aids in detoxification. Always brush in the direction of elimination, i.e. up the legs, up the arms, down the torso.

✓ **Kindness**
Routinely doing something kind for someone with no strings attached.

✓ **Bowel movements** Less than one bowel movement per day spells trouble.

Daily Progress Chart

Start Date _____ **Week #** _____

Item	1	2	3	4	5	6	7	Total
6-8 glasses pure water								
20-30 minutes of aerobic exercise								
3 servings fresh fruit								
5 servings fresh vegetables								
Alcohol-free								
Raw sugar free								
Nightshade free								
No fried or deep fried foods								
No soda pop								
Caffeine free								
Maintain 80/20 acid to alkaline ratio								
Dairy free								
White flour free								
Smoke free								
Fresh lemon juice								
Enzyme supplements								
Minimum of 2 tbs. of Omega 3/6 oils								
2 tablespoons granular lecithin								
One hour personal meditation								
Skin brushing for lymph stimulation								
One random act of kindness								
Minimum of one bowel movement								
Daily Total ->								Total

Daily Progress Chart

Start Date _____ **Week #** _____

Item	1	2	3	4	5	6	7	Total
6-8 glasses pure water								
20-30 minutes of aerobic exercise								
3 servings fresh fruit								
5 servings fresh vegetables								
Alcohol-free								
Raw sugar free								
Nightshade free								
No fried or deep fried foods								
No soda pop								
Caffeine free								
Maintain 80/20 acid to alkaline ratio								
Dairy free								
White flour free								
Smoke free								
Fresh lemon juice								
Enzyme supplements								
Minimum of 2 tbs. of Omega 3/6 oils								
2 tablespoons granular lecithin								
One hour personal meditation								
Skin brushing for lymph stimulation								
One random act of kindness								
Minimum of one bowel movement								
Daily Total ->								Total

Daily Progress Chart

Start Date _____ **Week #** _____

Item	1	2	3	4	5	6	7	Total
6-8 glasses pure water								
20-30 minutes of aerobic exercise								
3 servings fresh fruit								
5 servings fresh vegetables								
Alcohol-free								
Raw sugar free								
Nightshade free								
No fried or deep fried foods								
No soda pop								
Caffeine free								
Maintain 80/20 acid to alkaline ratio								
Dairy free								
White flour free								
Smoke free								
Fresh lemon juice								
Enzyme supplements								
Minimum of 2 tbs. of Omega 3/6 oils								
2 tablespoons granular lecithin								
One hour personal meditation								
Skin brushing for lymph stimulation								
One random act of kindness								
Minimum of one bowel movement								
Daily Total ->								Total

Daily Progress Chart

Start Date _____ **Week #** _____

Item	1	2	3	4	5	6	7	Total
6-8 glasses pure water								
20-30 minutes of aerobic exercise								
3 servings fresh fruit								
5 servings fresh vegetables								
Alcohol-free								
Raw sugar free								
Nightshade free								
No fried or deep fried foods								
No soda pop								
Caffeine free								
Maintain 80/20 acid to alkaline ratio								
Dairy free								
White flour free								
Smoke free								
Fresh lemon juice								
Enzyme supplements								
Minimum of 2 tbs. of Omega 3/6 oils								
2 tablespoons granular lecithin								
One hour personal meditation								
Skin brushing for lymph stimulation								
One random act of kindness								
Minimum of one bowel movement								
Daily Total ->								Total

Daily Progress Chart

Start Date _____ **Week #** _____

Item	1	2	3	4	5	6	7	Total
6-8 glasses pure water								
20-30 minutes of aerobic exercise								
3 servings fresh fruit								
5 servings fresh vegetables								
Alcohol-free								
Raw sugar free								
Nightshade free								
No fried or deep fried foods								
No soda pop								
Caffeine free								
Maintain 80/20 acid to alkaline ratio								
Dairy free								
White flour free								
Smoke free								
Fresh lemon juice								
Enzyme supplements								
Minimum of 2 tbs. of Omega 3/6 oils								
2 tablespoons granular lecithin								
One hour personal meditation								
Skin brushing for lymph stimulation								
One random act of kindness								
Minimum of one bowel movement								
Daily Total ->								Total

Daily Progress Chart

Start Date _____ **Week #** _____

Item	1	2	3	4	5	6	7	Total
6-8 glasses pure water								
20-30 minutes of aerobic exercise								
3 servings fresh fruit								
5 servings fresh vegetables								
Alcohol-free								
Raw sugar free								
Nightshade free								
No fried or deep fried foods								
No soda pop								
Caffeine free								
Maintain 80/20 acid to alkaline ratio								
Dairy free								
White flour free								
Smoke free								
Fresh lemon juice								
Enzyme supplements								
Minimum of 2 tbs. of Omega 3/6 oils								
2 tablespoons granular lecithin								
One hour personal meditation								
Skin brushing for lymph stimulation								
One random act of kindness								
Minimum of one bowel movement								
Daily Total ->								Total

Daily Progress Chart

Start Date _____ **Week #** _____

Item	1	2	3	4	5	6	7	Total
6-8 glasses pure water								
20-30 minutes of aerobic exercise								
3 servings fresh fruit								
5 servings fresh vegetables								
Alcohol-free								
Raw sugar free								
Nightshade free								
No fried or deep fried foods								
No soda pop								
Caffeine free								
Maintain 80/20 acid to alkaline ratio								
Dairy free								
White flour free								
Smoke free								
Fresh lemon juice								
Enzyme supplements								
Minimum of 2 tbs. of Omega 3/6 oils								
2 tablespoons granular lecithin								
One hour personal meditation								
Skin brushing for lymph stimulation								
One random act of kindness								
Minimum of one bowel movement								
Daily Total ->								Total

Daily Progress Chart

Start Date _____ **Week #** _____

Item	1	2	3	4	5	6	7	Total
6-8 glasses pure water								
20-30 minutes of aerobic exercise								
3 servings fresh fruit								
5 servings fresh vegetables								
Alcohol-free								
Raw sugar free								
Nightshade free								
No fried or deep fried foods								
No soda pop								
Caffeine free								
Maintain 80/20 acid to alkaline ratio								
Dairy free								
White flour free								
Smoke free								
Fresh lemon juice								
Enzyme supplements								
Minimum of 2 tbs. of Omega 3/6 oils								
2 tablespoons granular lecithin								
One hour personal meditation								
Skin brushing for lymph stimulation								
One random act of kindness								
Minimum of one bowel movement								
Daily Total ->								Total

Daily Progress Chart

Start Date _____ **Week #** _____

Item	1	2	3	4	5	6	7	Total
6-8 glasses pure water								
20-30 minutes of aerobic exercise								
3 servings fresh fruit								
5 servings fresh vegetables								
Alcohol-free								
Raw sugar free								
Nightshade free								
No fried or deep fried foods								
No soda pop								
Caffeine free								
Maintain 80/20 acid to alkaline ratio								
Dairy free								
White flour free								
Smoke free								
Fresh lemon juice								
Enzyme supplements								
Minimum of 2 tbs. of Omega 3/6 oils								
2 tablespoons granular lecithin								
One hour personal meditation								
Skin brushing for lymph stimulation								
One random act of kindness								
Minimum of one bowel movement								
Daily Total ->								Total

Daily Progress Chart

Start Date _____ **Week #** _____

Item	1	2	3	4	5	6	7	Total
6-8 glasses pure water								
20-30 minutes of aerobic exercise								
3 servings fresh fruit								
5 servings fresh vegetables								
Alcohol-free								
Raw sugar free								
Nightshade free								
No fried or deep fried foods								
No soda pop								
Caffeine free								
Maintain 80/20 acid to alkaline ratio								
Dairy free								
White flour free								
Smoke free								
Fresh lemon juice								
Enzyme supplements								
Minimum of 2 tbs. of Omega 3/6 oils								
2 tablespoons granular lecithin								
One hour personal meditation								
Skin brushing for lymph stimulation								
One random act of kindness								
Minimum of one bowel movement								
Daily Total ->								Total

142

Daily Progress Chart

Start Date _____ **Week #** _____

Item	1	2	3	4	5	6	7	Total
6-8 glasses pure water								
20-30 minutes of aerobic exercise								
3 servings fresh fruit								
5 servings fresh vegetables								
Alcohol-free								
Raw sugar free								
Nightshade free								
No fried or deep fried foods								
No soda pop								
Caffeine free								
Maintain 80/20 acid to alkaline ratio								
Dairy free								
White flour free								
Smoke free								
Fresh lemon juice								
Enzyme supplements								
Minimum of 2 tbs. of Omega 3/6 oils								
2 tablespoons granular lecithin								
One hour personal meditation								
Skin brushing for lymph stimulation								
One random act of kindness								
Minimum of one bowel movement								
Daily Total ->								Total

Daily Progress Chart

Start Date _____ **Week #** _____

Item	1	2	3	4	5	6	7	Total
6-8 glasses pure water								
20-30 minutes of aerobic exercise								
3 servings fresh fruit								
5 servings fresh vegetables								
Alcohol-free								
Raw sugar free								
Nightshade free								
No fried or deep fried foods								
No soda pop								
Caffeine free								
Maintain 80/20 acid to alkaline ratio								
Dairy free								
White flour free								
Smoke free								
Fresh lemon juice								
Enzyme supplements								
Minimum of 2 tbs. of Omega 3/6 oils								
2 tablespoons granular lecithin								
One hour personal meditation								
Skin brushing for lymph stimulation								
One random act of kindness								
Minimum of one bowel movement								
Daily Total ->								Total

Daily Progress Chart

Start Date _____ **Week #** _____

Item	1	2	3	4	5	6	7	Total
6-8 glasses pure water								
20-30 minutes of aerobic exercise								
3 servings fresh fruit								
5 servings fresh vegetables								
Alcohol-free								
Raw sugar free								
Nightshade free								
No fried or deep fried foods								
No soda pop								
Caffeine free								
Maintain 80/20 acid to alkaline ratio								
Dairy free								
White flour free								
Smoke free								
Fresh lemon juice								
Enzyme supplements								
Minimum of 2 tbs. of Omega 3/6 oils								
2 tablespoons granular lecithin								
One hour personal meditation								
Skin brushing for lymph stimulation								
One random act of kindness								
Minimum of one bowel movement								
Daily Total ->								Total

Daily Progress Chart

Start Date _____ **Week #** _____

Item	1	2	3	4	5	6	7	Total
6-8 glasses pure water								
20-30 minutes of aerobic exercise								
3 servings fresh fruit								
5 servings fresh vegetables								
Alcohol-free								
Raw sugar free								
Nightshade free								
No fried or deep fried foods								
No soda pop								
Caffeine free								
Maintain 80/20 acid to alkaline ratio								
Dairy free								
White flour free								
Smoke free								
Fresh lemon juice								
Enzyme supplements								
Minimum of 2 tbs. of Omega 3/6 oils								
2 tablespoons granular lecithin								
One hour personal meditation								
Skin brushing for lymph stimulation								
One random act of kindness								
Minimum of one bowel movement								
Daily Total ->								Total

Daily Progress Chart

Start Date _____ Week # _____

Item	1	2	3	4	5	6	7	Total
6-8 glasses pure water								
20-30 minutes of aerobic exercise								
3 servings fresh fruit								
5 servings fresh vegetables								
Alcohol-free								
Raw sugar free								
Nightshade free								
No fried or deep fried foods								
No soda pop								
Caffeine free								
Maintain 80/20 acid to alkaline ratio								
Dairy free								
White flour free								
Smoke free								
Fresh lemon juice								
Enzyme supplements								
Minimum of 2 tbs. of Omega 3/6 oils								
2 tablespoons granular lecithin								
One hour personal meditation								
Skin brushing for lymph stimulation								
One random act of kindness								
Minimum of one bowel movement								
Daily Total ->								Total

Daily Progress Chart

Start Date _____ **Week #** _____

Item	1	2	3	4	5	6	7	Total
6-8 glasses pure water								
20-30 minutes of aerobic exercise								
3 servings fresh fruit								
5 servings fresh vegetables								
Alcohol-free								
Raw sugar free								
Nightshade free								
No fried or deep fried foods								
No soda pop								
Caffeine free								
Maintain 80/20 acid to alkaline ratio								
Dairy free								
White flour free								
Smoke free								
Fresh lemon juice								
Enzyme supplements								
Minimum of 2 tbs. of Omega 3/6 oils								
2 tablespoons granular lecithin								
One hour personal meditation								
Skin brushing for lymph stimulation								
One random act of kindness								
Minimum of one bowel movement								
Daily Total ->								Total

148

Daily Progress Chart

Start Date _____ **Week #** _____

Item	1	2	3	4	5	6	7	Total
6-8 glasses pure water								
20-30 minutes of aerobic exercise								
3 servings fresh fruit								
5 servings fresh vegetables								
Alcohol-free								
Raw sugar free								
Nightshade free								
No fried or deep fried foods								
No soda pop								
Caffeine free								
Maintain 80/20 acid to alkaline ratio								
Dairy free								
White flour free								
Smoke free								
Fresh lemon juice								
Enzyme supplements								
Minimum of 2 tbs. of Omega 3/6 oils								
2 tablespoons granular lecithin								
One hour personal meditation								
Skin brushing for lymph stimulation								
One random act of kindness								
Minimum of one bowel movement								
Daily Total ->								Total

Daily Progress Chart

Start Date _____ **Week #** _____

Item	1	2	3	4	5	6	7	Total
6-8 glasses pure water								
20-30 minutes of aerobic exercise								
3 servings fresh fruit								
5 servings fresh vegetables								
Alcohol-free								
Raw sugar free								
Nightshade free								
No fried or deep fried foods								
No soda pop								
Caffeine free								
Maintain 80/20 acid to alkaline ratio								
Dairy free								
White flour free								
Smoke free								
Fresh lemon juice								
Enzyme supplements								
Minimum of 2 tbs. of Omega 3/6 oils								
2 tablespoons granular lecithin								
One hour personal meditation								
Skin brushing for lymph stimulation								
One random act of kindness								
Minimum of one bowel movement								
Daily Total ->								Total

Daily Progress Chart

Start Date _____ **Week #** _____

Item	1	2	3	4	5	6	7	Total
6-8 glasses pure water								
20-30 minutes of aerobic exercise								
3 servings fresh fruit								
5 servings fresh vegetables								
Alcohol-free								
Raw sugar free								
Nightshade free								
No fried or deep fried foods								
No soda pop								
Caffeine free								
Maintain 80/20 acid to alkaline ratio								
Dairy free								
White flour free								
Smoke free								
Fresh lemon juice								
Enzyme supplements								
Minimum of 2 tbs. of Omega 3/6 oils								
2 tablespoons granular lecithin								
One hour personal meditation								
Skin brushing for lymph stimulation								
One random act of kindness								
Minimum of one bowel movement								
Daily Total ->								Total

Daily Progress Chart

Start Date _____ **Week #** _____

Item	1	2	3	4	5	6	7	Total
6-8 glasses pure water								
20-30 minutes of aerobic exercise								
3 servings fresh fruit								
5 servings fresh vegetables								
Alcohol-free								
Raw sugar free								
Nightshade free								
No fried or deep fried foods								
No soda pop								
Caffeine free								
Maintain 80/20 acid to alkaline ratio								
Dairy free								
White flour free								
Smoke free								
Fresh lemon juice								
Enzyme supplements								
Minimum of 2 tbs. of Omega 3/6 oils								
2 tablespoons granular lecithin								
One hour personal meditation								
Skin brushing for lymph stimulation								
One random act of kindness								
Minimum of one bowel movement								
Daily Total ->								Total

Daily Progress Chart

Start Date _____ **Week #** _____

Item	1	2	3	4	5	6	7	Total
6-8 glasses pure water								
20-30 minutes of aerobic exercise								
3 servings fresh fruit								
5 servings fresh vegetables								
Alcohol-free								
Raw sugar free								
Nightshade free								
No fried or deep fried foods								
No soda pop								
Caffeine free								
Maintain 80/20 acid to alkaline ratio								
Dairy free								
White flour free								
Smoke free								
Fresh lemon juice								
Enzyme supplements								
Minimum of 2 tbs. of Omega 3/6 oils								
2 tablespoons granular lecithin								
One hour personal meditation								
Skin brushing for lymph stimulation								
One random act of kindness								
Minimum of one bowel movement								
Daily Total ->								Total

Daily Progress Chart

Start Date _____ **Week #** _____

Item	1	2	3	4	5	6	7	Total
6-8 glasses pure water								
20-30 minutes of aerobic exercise								
3 servings fresh fruit								
5 servings fresh vegetables								
Alcohol-free								
Raw sugar free								
Nightshade free								
No fried or deep fried foods								
No soda pop								
Caffeine free								
Maintain 80/20 acid to alkaline ratio								
Dairy free								
White flour free								
Smoke free								
Fresh lemon juice								
Enzyme supplements								
Minimum of 2 tbs. of Omega 3/6 oils								
2 tablespoons granular lecithin								
One hour personal meditation								
Skin brushing for lymph stimulation								
One random act of kindness								
Minimum of one bowel movement								
Daily Total ->								Total

Daily Progress Chart

Start Date _____ **Week #** _____

Item	1	2	3	4	5	6	7	Total
6-8 glasses pure water								
20-30 minutes of aerobic exercise								
3 servings fresh fruit								
5 servings fresh vegetables								
Alcohol-free								
Raw sugar free								
Nightshade free								
No fried or deep fried foods								
No soda pop								
Caffeine free								
Maintain 80/20 acid to alkaline ratio								
Dairy free								
White flour free								
Smoke free								
Fresh lemon juice								
Enzyme supplements								
Minimum of 2 tbs. of Omega 3/6 oils								
2 tablespoons granular lecithin								
One hour personal meditation								
Skin brushing for lymph stimulation								
One random act of kindness								
Minimum of one bowel movement								
Daily Total ->								Total

Daily Progress Chart

Start Date _____ **Week #** _____

Item	1	2	3	4	5	6	7	Total
6-8 glasses pure water								
20-30 minutes of aerobic exercise								
3 servings fresh fruit								
5 servings fresh vegetables								
Alcohol-free								
Raw sugar free								
Nightshade free								
No fried or deep fried foods								
No soda pop								
Caffeine free								
Maintain 80/20 acid to alkaline ratio								
Dairy free								
White flour free								
Smoke free								
Fresh lemon juice								
Enzyme supplements								
Minimum of 2 tbs. of Omega 3/6 oils								
2 tablespoons granular lecithin								
One hour personal meditation								
Skin brushing for lymph stimulation								
One random act of kindness								
Minimum of one bowel movement								
Daily Total ->								Total

Daily Progress Chart

Start Date _____ **Week #** _____

Item	1	2	3	4	5	6	7	Total
6-8 glasses pure water								
20-30 minutes of aerobic exercise								
3 servings fresh fruit								
5 servings fresh vegetables								
Alcohol-free								
Raw sugar free								
Nightshade free								
No fried or deep fried foods								
No soda pop								
Caffeine free								
Maintain 80/20 acid to alkaline ratio								
Dairy free								
White flour free								
Smoke free								
Fresh lemon juice								
Enzyme supplements								
Minimum of 2 tbs. of Omega 3/6 oils								
2 tablespoons granular lecithin								
One hour personal meditation								
Skin brushing for lymph stimulation								
One random act of kindness								
Minimum of one bowel movement								
Daily Total ->								Total

What is it about this that can work for you?

Once your diet has been altered to conform to the regimen, you cannot help but improve. Continuance of the regimen over a lengthy period of time will ensure that your body not only receives the nutrients it needs, but it also will be in a position to expel the toxins that keep you from naturally healing. Remember this: the body will heal itself if given the proper tools and nutrients. After all, your body is made mostly of water, nutrients, and oxygen. If you degrade any of those, degeneration follows. Drinking no water means no replenishment of life force in your cells. Consuming degraded foods means depriving your cells of live food, the very essence of your being. Breathing poor quality air means less exchange of nutrients (energy) at the cellular level.

On the other hand, drinking lots of good water will produce the healthy cellular activity you need. Consuming high quality live foods ensures proper nutrients are available for rebuilding. Breathing good air and exercising provides essential oxygen for the transfer of nutrients to grow healthy cells, plus every healthy function in the body needs oxygen.

The Participant vs. the Drifter

Imagine what the health differences are between the two types of people in the chart below. Imagine how their relative health status grows further and further apart as time marches on. Then imagine the attitude they have when confronted with the necessity of making changes, many considered drastic by their standards.

Chances are that #1 does not have psoriasis in the first place. Ninety-six percent of #2 people don't have psoriasis regardless, because only 3-4 percent of humanity has it, and you are one of them. #2 people die of heart disease, cancer and stroke instead and don't think that they don't, because that's exactly what's happening in today's world.

The most pathetic excuse offered by too many people trying to justify their horrible lifestyles is "my grandfather smoked and drank until he was 95 and wasn't sick a day in his life". The missing information in this scenario is that their grandfather lived off the land, smoked real tobacco (not deadly chemicals) and drank for his health, not for recreation. These folks are not their grandfathers, and too much has changed for that to work anymore.

#1 Health Conscious Participant	#2 Drifter Takes it as it comes
Healthy home meal fixer	Regular restaurant eater
Fruit & vegetable eater	Eats little or none
6-8 glasses of water daily	Doesn't like water
Drinks herbal teas	Drinks coffee all day
Exercises daily	Couch potato
Body fat index good	Obese or overweight
Never touches pop	Drinks several pop a day
Avoids sugar	Loves desserts & candy
Non-smoker	Smoker
Takes time to relax	Social animal, never stops
Eats little meat	Loves steak & potatoes
Drinks a little wine	Regularly has beer, liquor
Plays sports	Watches sports on TV
Monitors own health	Relies on doctor for info

In order for you to heal, you need to become that #1 person. This might be a simple choice to make, but the work is not always so simple. This is precisely where the majority of people step off the program due to their unwillingness to roll up their sleeves and just do it. Whether they consider the sacrifice to be too great, or stresses keep them in a perpetual state of procrastination, it is obvious that their priorities are not clear enough for them to go forward. The other most regrettable factor is that their doctor has hexed them into believing that there is no way out. People tend to accept what the 'authorities' tell them, either consciously or subconsciously. This must be overcome before starting on your healing. Hopefully there is enough background information in this book to finally convince you that the establishment has misinformed you, and you can put it all behind you once and for all.

What are you willing to do to heal your psoriasis?

Dr. Phil McGraw wrote the bestseller 'Self Matters', a book that should be read by everyone with psoriasis to help with the emotional side of the disorder. In it, Dr. Phil, as he is affectionately known, explains the concept of 'locus of control'. Locus of control is the degree to which you attribute your health to internal responsibilities as compared to chance. If you have a high attribution to chance, your healing will be made that much more difficult.

Dr. Phil says,
"If you have little or no belief or trust in yourself or anything else, you will probably not put any faith in any health-related resource. You may not see any point in changing your diet or quitting smoking. Chance is a self-concept of *powerlessness*: You see no purpose in discipline and therefore have zero motivation to change."

What's *your* bottom line? Are you prepared yet to do some work to change your life? The statistics are grim for anyone who is not wholeheartedly involved in their own healing, who has not 'internalized' responsibility. The unwillingness of the majority of psoriatics to participate, coupled with attributing their condition to 'outside' sources, explains why the proven fundamentals of healing psoriasis are not on the front pages of the medical journals. Doctors do not have the time or the inclination to baby-sit people, so the 'no cure' paradigm persists to this day. Because the vast majority of people still do not heal for the above reasons, the typical doctor does not want to be implicated in another failure, and who would blame them with a 90% failure rate. As has just been explained throughout this chapter, it is all but a foregone conclusion that you will heal if you take all the steps. No half-measures will do. This takes time as indeed it took time for your body to develop psoriasis in the first place, yet nothing can stop you if you have the right attitude and preparedness.

Start, and don't stop until you succeed. It's up to you.

160

Reality Check #12

If you've read this far in the book, you perhaps realize not only what you have been through all this time with your psoriasis, but also what you're up against. Maybe you can accept the fact that you've never really given it your full effort, or *maybe you didn't even know what to do until now*. It will be a major turn of events in your life when you reach that point in time when you are finally READY to take action – no matter what it takes – until you are healed.

Are you at that point?

Chapter 13

How you can Help Yourself & Others

A final wish is that you enjoy your life in the knowledge that you have the power to make effective changes to your being; that you will be able to keep the 3 benchmarks of healing in mind as you continue to improve over the months to come:

- Detoxification
- Transformation
- Control

While conventional medical wisdom teaches the vast majority of the population that there is no known cause and no known cure for psoriasis, others of us know differently. For us, it is important on a human level to share what we have learned, especially having proven it to ourselves.

If you are willing to move outside of your comfort zone you will find not only complete relief from your psoriasis, but a fuller life. Exploring solutions to the problem from every angle possible is very important. It also runs through the course of this work that it takes mind, body and spirit together to be well. It is fundamental to know in your heart that psoriasis can indeed be healed, even though your own practical knowledge of that may have to come later. The human being is complex, so this must be kept in mind at all times in order not to rule out any special strategy peculiar to yourself.

No matter what your experience with psoriasis has been, your willingness to participate in your own disorder can and will make a significant difference in terms of a healing. This is not conjecture, but the real experience of many professionals trained in the field of natural medicine. Far from a fringe idea, the medical world is realizing that knowledge of self is a powerful force in healing, and psoriasis is certainly one of them.

Now, the problem is that people are not aware of choices. They visit the doctor, get the prescription along with the 'medical hex' (no known cure), and go home to suffer for years. If ever there was a need for people to take ownership of a condition, this is it. Once you have experienced the relief that comes from doing the work, it is incumbent upon you to let others know about it. Ninety-five percent of the estimated 25 million people with psoriasis in North America will never hear of full natural healing unless someone outside the medical community tells them about it. That means you and I.

"When you have been given a gift of great value, you are obligated to share it over and over."
- Old Chinese proverb

Without actually doing much of anything, you have the power to positively affect the lives of others. Just imagine how simple it would be to mention to someone else who is suffering with psoriasis that there is a website, or some information they can visit to help them escape. The word 'escape' is meant in the literal sense. Having learned of this new information, and especially once you prove it to yourself, you have quite literally escaped from the clutches of medical paralytic thinking as well as from the trap line of the pharmaceutical companies.

The organization known as PCI (Psoriasis Connection International) began in 1998 with an Internet presence to be able to reach more people outside of traditional medical circles. This has been successful, but only as a start. There are millions more people ready to hear about 'another way'. Pass along **psconnect.com** to them so they can be in touch too.

Keep in touch with the website yourself, because as a purchaser of this book, you are entitled to the ongoing support we have available on this website – indefinitely.

First, help yourself. Afterwards, or simultaneously, help others to find the information that will release them.

No more or less can you do. Best Wishes.

Resources

Internet

The websites below are unrelated to this publication and have no connection to this work. They are, however, compatible in philosophy with the natural healing principles discussed in this book. Material covered on these websites is presented by the owners of the websites, and is their responsibility. Having said that, they are highly recommended as credible sources of good information to help with your general understanding of health.

Dr. Joseph Mercola
www.mercola.com
Free weekly subscription to health articles, plus search database.

Dr. Andrew Weil
www.drweil.com
Alternative/natural medicine

Dr. Deepak Chopra
www.chopra.com
Ayurvedic medicine, meditation techniques, and more.

Dr. Udo Erasmus
www.udoerasmus.com
Essential Fatty Acids – Explanation & Ordering Source

Chem-tox.com
Website dedicated to health disorders caused by chemicals & pesticides
www.chem-tox.com

The Psoriasis Connection (PCI Support)
Ongoing, online support by virtue of owning this book.
www.psconnect.com

Suggested Books for Further Reading
(Alphabetical)

Diet & Nutrition – a Holistic Approach
Dr. Rudolph Ballentine, M.D.
ISBN 0-89389-048-0

Fats That Heal, Fats That Kill
Dr. Udo Erasmus
ISBN 0-920470-38-6

Gastro-intestinal Health
Steven R. Peikin, M.D.
ISBN 0-06-095318-7

Hard to Swallow – the Truth About Food Additives
Doris Sarjeant
ISBN 0-920470-47-5

Healing Psoriasis – the Natural Alternative
Dr. John Pagano
ISBN 0-9628847-0-7

Healing with Whole Foods
Paul Pritchard
ISBN 1-55643-220-8

Intuitive Eating
Dr. Humbart Santillo
ISBN 0-934252-27-0

Leaky Gut Syndrome
Elizabeth Lipski
ISBN 0-879838-24-8

Nutrition & Physical Degeneration
Weston A. Price, D.D.S.
ISBN 0-87983-816-7

Optimal Digestion – New Strategies for Achieving Digestive Health
Trent Nichols, M.D. and Nancy Faass, MSW, MPH
ISBN 0-380-80498-0

The 22 Non-negotiable Laws of Wellness
Greg Anderson
ISBN 0-06-251299-4

The Chemistry of Success: Six Secrets of Peak Performance
Susan Lark, M.D. & James Richards, MBA
ISBN 1-57959-501-4

Winning the War Against Immune Disorders & Allergies
Ellen W. Cutler, D.C.
ISBN 0-7668-0059-8

Yeast Connection and the Woman
William G. Crook, M.D.
ISBN 0-933478-22-4 [Note: good for men too]

Your Body's Many Cries for Water
F. Batmanghelidj, M.D.
ISBN 0-9629942-3-5

Sources of Supply

Essential Oils (EFA's)
Purchase at your health food store.
Research Dr. Udo Erasmus' website at
www.udoerasmus.com

Whole, Raw Fruit & Vegetable Supplementation
In capsules, sugar & salt removed, enzymes included.
Vegetables: carrots, spinach, parsley, beets, kale, broccoli, cabbage, tomato, barley, and oats.
Fruits: apples, oranges, pineapple, cranberries peaches, acerola cherries, papaya.
Email **support@psconnect.com** for the contact name of the nearest source of whole food supplements.

Special Herbal Teas etc.
Purchase at your health food store.
Alternatively, Association for Research & Enlightenment
www.are-cayce.com

Granular Lecithin
Purchase at your health food store.

Colon Cleansing Programs
Purchase at your health food store.

Index